Our Love Affair with Drugs

Our Love Affair with Drugs: The History, the Science, the Politics

Jerrold Winter, PhD

Professor of Pharmacology and Toxicology
Jacobs School of Medicine and Biomedical Sciences
University at Buffalo

OXFORD
UNIVERSITY PRESS

OXFORD
UNIVERSITY PRESS

Oxford University Press is a department of the University of Oxford. It furthers the University's objective of excellence in research, scholarship, and education by publishing worldwide. Oxford is a registered trade mark of Oxford University Press in the UK and certain other countries.

Published in the United States of America by Oxford University Press
198 Madison Avenue, New York, NY 10016, United States of America.

Library of Congress Cataloging-in-Publication Data
Names: Winter, Jerrold, author.
Title: Our love affair with drugs: the history, the science, the politics / Jerrold Winter.
Description: New York, NY : Oxford University Press, [2020] |
Includes bibliographical references and index.
Identifiers: LCCN 2019014952| ISBN 9780190051464 (hardback) |
ISBN 9780190051471 (updf) | ISBN 9780190051488 (epub)
Subjects: | MESH: Psychotropic Drugs | Central Nervous System Agents |
Substance-Related Disorders—prevention & control | Public Policy |
Drug and Narcotic Control
Classification: LCC RM315 | NLM QV 77.2 | DDC 615.7/88—dc23
LC record available at https://lccn.loc.gov/2019014952

1 3 5 7 9 8 6 4 2

Printed by Integrated Books International, United States of America

To Barbara

CONTENTS

CONTENTS

PREFACE

This book is about psychoactive drugs. For me, the adjective *psychoactive* has a touch of pretention about it. We might better say that these are simply drugs that in various ways influence the way our brains function. Manifestations of their influence on the brain are quite varied. There may be the comfort provided by opioids to those who are dying or in pain or, in everyday life, the surge of contentment for the users of caffeine, nicotine, heroin, alcohol, or marijuana upon the taking of their drug of choice. Turning to the more exotic, a drug such as LSD may alter the way the world looks to us; it may even inspire thoughts of God. All of this and more is encompassed by *psychoactive*; the term, I must admit, has the virtue of brevity and I will use it often, but we should ever keep in mind the enormous complexity of our brains and the actions of drugs upon them. Adding to the purely scientific questions which confront us are the ways in which our society chooses to respond to the presence of psychoactive drugs. Should they be banned and their users sent to prison, tolerated as a reflection of man's eternal search for an escape from anxiety, pain, and the monotony of daily life, or celebrated as therapeutically useful agents?

This book is an attempt to bring order and genuine understanding to the thousands of bits of information which swirl about us concerning psychoactive drugs. These come to us from newspapers, magazines, television, social media, the Internet, and in everyday conversation with family and friends. To accomplish this end, we must strive to attain total perspective. The rise of the Internet has made achieving such perspective both easier and more difficult. Easier because an enormous store of information is readily at hand; a Google search today will turn up 462 million hits for LSD, including offers to sell us the drug. But our striving for total perspective is made more difficult because, as we are inundated with information from all sides, we may become, not informed, but more confused.

In commenting on those who write for the general reader about psychoactive drugs, Daniel Kunitz, a noted editor and author, said that "the grail is a comprehensive tome that would reveal the secrets of all drugs and would stand as the last, totalizing word on the subject." Alas, *Our Love Affair with Drugs: The History, the Science, the Politics* is not that book. Indeed, the Kunitz goal has never been reached nor is it ever to be reached, for there can be no last word on an ever-changing subject. There is no place for dogma in writing of these drugs. What we believe today is only the best approximation of truth based on what has come before. We must ever be prepared to alter our beliefs as Nature's secrets are revealed by the methods of science.

This book is divided into nine chapters, the middle seven of which are concerned with individual drugs or drug classes. It is my hope that these chapters are made intelligible by the contents of chapter 1, in which I introduce the reader to that branch of medical science called pharmacology. Central to that introduction is the concept of the drug receptor and the phenomena of drug tolerance, physical dependence, and addiction. The middle seven chapters can be read pretty much in any order. A reader with a particular interest in hallucinogens may wish to start with chapter 7. However, I do recommend that chapter 1 be read first as it will provide a basis of understanding for all that follows.

The contents of this book are largely factual, for example, the consequences of an overdose with heroin or a heart attack following the use of cocaine or methamphetamine or evidence of benefit provided to epileptic children by derivatives of marijuana or by ecstasy (MDMA) for a veteran suffering from posttraumatic stress disorder. I will, however, insert my personal opinions from time to time but, in all instances, will strive to identify them as such. These personal opinions are most evident in the final chapter, which deals with our war on drugs and the tools with which we have chosen to fight it.

I welcome the reader to join me on what I hope is an informative and even sometimes an enjoyable trip.

ACKNOWLEDGMENTS

There are many to whom I owe thanks. Among those who will remain nameless are the staff of the Health Sciences Library (HSL) of the University at Buffalo. The superb holdings of the HSL have provided me with many pleasurable hours and form the backbone of this book. The conversion of their journal collection to electronic form has saved me many trips to the HSL but unfortunately has diminished my personal contact with the staff. The medical literature is, of course, entirely the work of countless scientists, physicians, and scholars; some have been named, many more have not. To each I am indebted.

I thank the students who for a time shared my laboratory and who are now my mentors. From them I have learned far more than I taught. It was a privilege to know them all. In the writing of the present book, I am particularly indebted to Katherine R. Bonson, PhD, Scott Helsley, MD, PhD, David J. McCann, PhD, and Chad J. Reissig, PhD. Special thanks go to Mireille M. Meyerhoefer, MD, PhD, who read each chapter as it was completed and offered valuable criticism.

My colleagues in the Department of Pharmacology and Toxicology of the Jacobs School of Medicine and Biomedical Sciences of the University at Buffalo have been unstinting in sharing with me their profound knowledge of drugs. Thanks go to Margarita Dubocovich, PhD, and David Dietz, PhD, who chaired the Department during the time that this book was in progress. David Nichols, PhD, and Rick Strassman, MD, both of whom have been major contributors to our understanding of psychoactive drugs, offered helpful comments regarding my chapter on hallucinogens. Rick Doblin, PhD, kindly corrected my account of his crusade to bring MDMA into clinical use. Daphne Lloyd-Alders, MD, PhD, and Howard Chambers, MD, PhD, provided support whenever it was needed.

This project would not have been completed without the superb professionalism of Jeremy Lewis and Bronwyn Geyer of the Oxford University Press. The assistance of Raj Suthan and Leslie Anglin is much appreciated.

Finally, I will be forever grateful to Andy Ross of the Andy Ross Literary Agency for being the first to have had faith in this undertaking.

My children, Anne, Jerrold, Jr., Kurt, and Jessica, have endured decades of my talk about drugs, and I thank them for their forbearance. The book is dedicated to Barbara, my wife of 59 years and a constant source of encouragement.

Our Love Affair with Drugs

CHAPTER 1

ℭ

Pharmacology

The Science of Drugs

Aldous Huxley once said that man was a pharmacologist before he was a farmer.[1] Although written records rarely go back more than 5,000 or 6,000 years, there is reason to believe that humans did indeed experience the effects of a variety of drugs much earlier, perhaps even before the rise of agriculture some 12,000 years ago in the Nile Valley. Likely drugs available to the ancients include opiates, cocaine, tetrahydrocannabinol, cathinone, and numerous hallucinogens. But these were drugs in their crude natural forms: the opium poppy, coca leaves, hemp, khat, and a variety of other plant sources. Identification of pure chemicals and a science of drugs was much slower in coming.

Pharmacology had to wait for the rise early in the 19th century of organic chemistry, largely in Germany, and physiology, chiefly in France and England.[2] Pharmacology was born of the marriage of these two disciplines. Signifying its maturation in this country, the first department of pharmacology was established at Johns Hopkins University School of Medicine in 1893. Today, pharmacology is taught as a basic medical science, along with anatomy, pathology, physiology, biochemistry, and microbiology, to every medical student.

Each of the drugs I mentioned earlier will be discussed in detail in the chapters that follow, but before we do this we need a basic pharmacological vocabulary and a little knowledge of how drugs act. Pharmacology deals with the interaction of chemicals with a living system: the human body.

Our Love Affair with Drugs: The History, the Science, the Politics. Jerrold Winter, Oxford University Press (2020). © Jerrold Winter.
DOI: 10.1093/oso/9780190051464.001.0001

Although drugs act on every element of the body, we will be most interested in that most complex of organs, the brain.

DRUG MOLECULES AND OUR BRAINS

We are aware that a drug has acted upon our brains by the effects that it produces. These effects may be as direct and unequivocal as vomiting after apomorphine or convulsing after strychnine. These effects may be of such subtlety as to inspire poetry or to stimulate thoughts of God. Diffuse, relaxed pleasure or orgasmic high; tranquility or terror: Drugs can produce any of these reactions and more. Some drugs may even inspire us to love our fellow man. And in every instance the effects of a drug are colored and made still more complex by the structure and past experience and current state of the brain upon which it acts. No wonder that humans throughout their history have been fascinated by such chemicals.

Most readers of this book have had ample opportunity to experience the effects of numerous drugs over their lifetime. For example, I daily ingest what I like to call a "geriatric cocktail" aimed at staving off cardiovascular problems. This consists of metoprolol (Lopressor), atorvastatin (Lipitor), ramipril (Altace), aspirin, and hydrochlorothiazide. When it comes to drugs acting on my brain, I have caffeine in the form of Coke or Pepsi or chocolate, alcohol in beer and wine or, on a good day, a margarita or two, and, if my sciatica is acting up, a modest dose of hydrocodone, an opioid, in combination with acetaminophen (Vicodin). In listing these drugs, you may have noticed that I said metoprolol (Lopressor), atorvastatin (Lipitor), ramipril (Altace), and hydrocodone in combination with acetaminophen (Vicodin). The capitalized name is a trade or proprietary name; the other is the generic name. The trade name is the one most often heard by patients, at least until the patent on the drug runs out and a generic form is available. Most of the drugs we will be talking about will be addressed by their generic name, but if a drug such as fluoxetine is well known by its trade name Prozac, I will use that as well.

The basic unit of every drug is the molecule, the smallest particle of the drug that retains all of the drug's properties. There are lots of them. The modest doses of the five drugs in my daily geriatric cocktail alone contain about 5×10^{20} molecules; that's 5 followed by 20 zeros. How in the world do they know where to go? I know where I *want* them to go: metoprolol, atorvastatin, ramipril, and aspirin to one or another element of my circulatory system; hydrochlorothiazide to my kidneys; caffeine, alcohol, and hydrocodone to my brain. But the fact is that they don't know where to go—once in the bloodstream, my drugs, with few exceptions, bathe virtually every cell and organ in my body. This does not mean that they act everywhere in my body.

DRUG RECEPTORS

In most instances a drug produces its desired effects by attaching itself to a structure of the cell called the receptor; receptors can be very selective, responding only to certain drugs and ignoring the rest. For example, opiates, about which much more will be said in chapter 2, reach receptors in the brain and spinal cord to dampen our experience of pain. But there are other opiate receptors. Some are in the gut and, when acted upon, can cause constipation.

Although the slowing of bowel activity by opiates does not strike fear as does addiction, constipation can be a major problem, especially in the elderly. After being treated with an opiate for postsurgical pain, the late comedian Robin Williams said he felt the need for a turd exorcism. More ominously, there are opiate receptors in a primitive area of the brain, the medulla oblongata. When opiates act on these receptors, the activity of the medulla is suppressed; breathing is slowed and may stop entirely. Death is the endpoint. Hardly a day goes by that we are not made aware by the media of this pharmacological fact. The death of Prince in 2016 at the hands of fentanyl, an especially potent opiate, was a much publicized and lamented but not unusual example.[3]

The concept of the receptor is fundamental to an understanding of drugs, and I will invoke it repeatedly in the chapters to follow. However, in preparing to talk about a variety of drugs with disparate mechanisms of action, I want to provide three additional definitions that are particularly relevant to the drugs acting on my brain and to which I will make frequent reference. These are for drug tolerance, physical dependence, and addiction. Morphine, the drug that remains the gold standard for the relief of severe pain, nicely illustrates the phenomena.

DRUG TOLERANCE AND PHYSICAL DEPENDENCE

Let us imagine that I suffer from metastatic cancer. My physician prescribes morphine, and the pain-relieving effects are wonderful. But, over time, in order to maintain analgesia, it is necessary to increase the amount of morphine that I receive. It is now said that I have become tolerant to morphine.

Blessedly, that tolerance can be overcome with increasing doses of the drug. I may, after a few months, receive on a daily basis a quantity of morphine that would have killed me prior to my development of tolerance.

Tolerance, in and of itself, is benign. On the other hand, if I am a user of illicit cocaine or heroin, other drugs to which a high degree of tolerance develops, tolerance presents a problem. To acquire larger doses requires more money. For those not blessed with wealth, available sources of more money may involve theft, robbery, or prostitution.

During the period that I am treated with increasing doses of morphine for my cancer pain, my brain is undergoing adaptive changes in addition to tolerance. Surprisingly, I am totally unaware that these adaptations have taken place. Only upon abruptly stopping my morphine are they manifest. Taken together, the constellation of signs and symptoms that results is called the withdrawal syndrome or abstinence syndrome. I am now said to be physically dependent on morphine.

In the physically dependent state, so long as the direct effects of the drug and the compensatory changes in my brain are in rough balance, nothing very remarkable happens. If I upset that balance by suddenly depriving myself of morphine, the fact my brain has been altered by the drug will quickly be evident. Put another way, after physical dependence has developed, the continued present of morphine is required for normal function. But, so long as the drug of dependence is provided, I will not experience withdrawal. As we will see later, avoidance of the abstinence syndrome can become a powerful motivator for the continued use of a drug. A full discussion of the morphine abstinence syndrome will be given in chapter 2.

Tolerance and physical dependence are invariable pharmacological phenomena. They have nothing to do with willpower or your moral character. They certainly have nothing to do with the law. Every human, indeed every living animal going far down the evolutionary scale, will develop physical dependence when exposed to an appropriate drug for an appropriate period of time. In treating my hypothetical cancer pain in a perfectly acceptable medical fashion, it is quite likely that I will become physically dependent upon morphine. Addiction is another matter.

ADDICTION

Before I provide you with the definition of *addiction* which I favor and which I will use throughout this book, we need to understand that there is no universally accepted definition. The situation is such that 40 years ago a committee of experts suggested that we get rid of the term as being ill-defined and unhelpful. Well, it didn't go away, and it will not go away, and we must face the fact that ambiguity and misunderstanding concerning addiction prevail at all levels of society. For this reason, any time we encounter anyone trying to tell us something about "addiction," whether it be labeling a person as an "addict," speaking of a drug said to induce addiction, or suggesting a means to treat addiction, we need first to establish what they mean by the word. Humpty Dumpty's dictum to Alice, "When *I* use a word—it means just what I choose it to mean—neither more nor less," will not satisfy us.

Let us begin with two authoritative definitions of addiction. The first comes to us from the Federation of State Medical Boards of the United States: "Addiction is a primary, chronic, neurobiological disease, with genetic, psychosocial, and environmental factors influencing its development and manifestations. It is characterized by behaviors that include impaired control over drug use, craving, compulsive use, and continued use despite harm."[4]

The second definition is provided by the American Association for Addiction Medicine (AAAM): "Addiction is a primary, chronic disease of brain reward, motivation, memory, and related circuitry. Dysfunction in these circuits leads to characteristic biological, psychological, social and spiritual manifestations. This is reflected in an individual pathologically pursuing reward and/or relief by substance use and other behaviors."[5] The Society provides an alphabetic mnemonic: inability to *A*bstain, impairment in *B*ehavioral control, *C*raving for drugs or rewarding experiences, *D*iminished recognition of significant problems, and a dysfunctional *E*motional response.

This concept of addiction as a chronic disease of the brain,[6] and thus possibly amenable to medical treatment, is antithetical to many who regard addiction as a moral failure, a condition we bring voluntarily upon ourselves. Given these uncertainties, I prefer a purely operational definition such as that provided by Alan Leshner, a former director of the National Institute on Drug Abuse, the primary funding agency for addiction research in the United States: Addiction is the behavioral state of compulsive, uncontrollable drug craving and seeking.[7]

I would amend Dr. Leshner's definition only to add that the drug of addiction must do harm to the individual. For example, caffeine is a drug that induces physical dependence; the abstinence syndrome is characterized by anxiety, insomnia, and headache. Most of us have known some who surely do compulsively crave and seek the drug but, because caffeine does no harm except in massive doses, we do not label the users, habitual coffee drinkers for example, as drug addicts. Alcoholism, on the other hand, completely fits our definition of addiction. Not only is there compulsive drug craving and seeking, but the drug harms the individual in multiple ways, including physical damage to the liver and other organs as well as inducing recurrent social or interpersonal problems.

DRUG-INDUCED PLEASURE/AVOIDANCE
OF WITHDRAWAL

As we will see in discussing the drugs we love in the chapters that follow, there are two major factors in the continued use of a drug of addiction. The first, often overlooked by those who oppose the use of any psychoactive drugs, is the fact that these drugs can bring us pleasure. This can take the form of the euphoria induced by a drug such as cocaine, the relaxation following an alcoholic drink or a deep drag on a nicotine or marijuana cigarette, the mystical state induced by a hallucinogen, or the relief of pain in our lives, whether that pain be psychic or physical.

The second major factor influencing the compulsive use of an addictive drug is avoidance of a withdrawal syndrome. Just as drug tolerance has different implications for the patient chronically treated for pain compared with the illicit user, so too does physical dependence. A cancer or postsurgical patient physically dependent on morphine and no longer in need of the drug can slowly be weaned off of the drug with minimal discomfort and no risk of addiction. In contrast, the morphine or alcohol addict must each day face the prospect of desperate illness; for him the avoidance of the abstinence syndrome provides a powerful incentive for continued use of the drug. To paraphrase Thomas Hardy, once you have been tormented by the withdrawal syndrome, mere relief becomes delight.

Past thinking about physical dependence and its role in addiction was based almost exclusively on the abstinence syndromes peculiar to opiates, drugs such as morphine and heroin, as will be discussed in chapter 2, and the depressant drugs of chapter 5, especially alcohol and the barbiturates. The syndromes differ in detail, but both are quite dramatic; abrupt withdrawal of alcohol can even be life-threatening. Then along came cocaine.

PHYSICAL VERSUS PSYCHOLOGICAL DEPENDENCE

Fifty years ago it was said that there was no abstinence syndrome, that is, no physical dependence, following chronic cocaine use, and as a result, cocaine would be a negligible factor in drug misuse. Indeed, one writer opined that there is no such thing as cocaine addiction.[8] Yet, in 2014, it was estimated that there were 1.5 million regular users of cocaine in the United States, with nearly a million meeting accepted psychiatric criteria for dependence or abuse. In 2017, there were more than 14,000 deaths involving cocaine.[9] The drug cartels are well aware of cocaine's appeal for many Americans; in 2017, Colombia alone produced 1,500 tons of the drug with most destined for the United States.[10]

How are we to rationalize this behavioral state of compulsive, uncontrollable cocaine craving and seeking which does harm to the individual, thus fully meeting our definition of addiction, but in the absence of physical dependence of the classical type? The explanation offered was the notion of *psychological dependence*. For example, smokers of cigarettes and users of cocaine were said to be merely psychologically dependent and not really addicted to nicotine and cocaine; these were *soft* drugs and not to be compared with *hard* drugs able to induce physical dependence of the kind seen in heroin addicts or alcoholics. American tobacco companies were particularly emphatic in their denial that nicotine is a drug that leads to both physical dependence and addiction.

What has changed is that we are now willing to accept as a withdrawal syndrome the irritability of the smoker denied his nicotine and the depression of a cokehead without a line to snort and the craving of both for a fix.[11] And this is as it should be; the notion that compulsion to use a drug is "just in your mind" forgets the wise remark of Susanna Kaysen that "a lot of mind is brain."[12] Put more formally, the rebound of compensatory homeostatic adjustments that manifest as anxiety, irritability, depression, or craving for a drug such as nicotine or cocaine are as real and as compelling for the nicotine or cocaine addict as are the aches, gooseflesh, and nausea of heroin withdrawal for the junkie. With the acceptance of the hypothesis that all human subjective states have a neurochemical basis, the notion of psychological dependence and artificial distinctions between hard and soft drugs may be discarded; addiction and its ability to control human behavior should be our focus. Smokers of nicotine cigarettes are as addicted as any heroin addict. Indeed, on a statistical basis, the heroin addict is more likely to escape his addiction.

In the chapters that follow, we will repeatedly revisit the concept of the drug receptor and our definitions of drug tolerance, physical dependence, and addiction as they apply to the drugs we love.

NOTES

1. Huxley A (1958) *Collected Essays*. New York: Harper & Brothers.
2. Holmstedt B, Liljestrand G (1963) *Readings in Pharmacology*. London: Pergamon Press.
3. Winter JC (2016) What addiction really means. www.slate.com/articles/health_ and_science/medical/examiner/2016/05/prince
4. Federation of State Medical Boards of the United States (2005) Model policy for the use of controlled substances for the treatment of pain. *J Pain Palliat Care Pharmacother* 19(2):73–78.
5. American Society of Addiction Medicine (2011) Definition of addiction. www.asam.irg/resources/definition-of-addiction
6. Volkow ND, Goob GF, McLellan AT (2016) Neurobiological advances from the brain disease model of addiction. *N Eng J Med* 374(4):363–371.
7. Leshner AI (1997) Addiction is a brain disease, and it matters. *Science* 278:45–47.
8. Ashley A (1975) *Cocaine: Its History, Use, and Effects*. New York: St. Martin's Press.
9. National Institute on Drug Abuse (2018) Overdose death rates. https:// www.drugabuse.gov/related-topics/trends-statistics/overdose-death-rates
10. United Nations Office on Drugs and Crime (2018) Coca crops in Colombia at all-time high. https://www.unodc.org/unodc/en/frontpage/2018/September/coca-crops-in-colombia-at-all-time-high--unodc-report-finds.html
11. Winter JC (1998) The re-demonizing of marijuana. *Pharm News* 5(3):22–27.
12. Kaysen S (1993) *Girl Interrupted*. New York: Vintage Books.

CHAPTER 2

☙

Opioids

God's Own Medicine

Albert Schweitzer called pain "a more terrible lord of mankind than even death." Thus, it is not surprising that humans have from the earliest times attempted to identify plants which might provide pain relief. *The Odyssey* by Homer provides a mythic account of the use of one such agent.

> Then Helen, daughter of Zeus, took other counsel. Straightaway she cast into the wine of which they were drinking a drug to quit all pain and strife, and bring forgetfulness of every ill. Whoso should drink this down, when it is mingled in the bowl, would not in the course of that day let a tear fall down over his cheeks, no, not though his mother and father should lie there dead . . . Such cunning drugs had the daughter of Zeus, drugs of healing, which Polydamna, the wife of Thor, had given her, a woman of Egypt, for there the earth, the giver of grain, bears the greatest store of drugs . . .[1]

More than a century ago, it was suggested by Oswald Schmiedeberg, a German scientist regarded by many as the father of modern pharmacology, that the drug to which Homer refers is opium for "no other natural product on the whole earth calls forth in man such a psychical blunting as the one described."[2] When today, in the fields of Afghanistan or Turkey or India, the seed capsule of the opium poppy, *Papaver somniferum*, is pierced, a milky fluid oozes from it which, when dried, is opium.

Our Love Affair with Drugs: The History, the Science, the Politics. Jerrold Winter, Oxford University Press (2020). © Jerrold Winter.
DOI: 10.1093/oso/9780190051464.001.0001

Virginia Berridge, in her elegant history of opium in England, tells us that the effects of opium on the human mind have probably been known for about 6,000 years and that opium had an honored place in Greek, Roman, and Arabic medicine.[3] I will not dwell on that ancient history but will instead jump ahead to the 17th century by which time opium had gained wide use in European medicine.

Writing in 1680, Thomas Sydenham, a British physician, said this: "Among the remedies it has pleased Almighty God to give to man to relieve his sufferings, none is so universal and so efficacious."[4] Sydenham's favored form of opium was a solution in alcohol, a combination which came to be called laudanum. In addition to the relief of pain, opium was employed against dysentery, asthma, uncontrollable cough, fever, and a variety of other ailments; even diabetes was an indication for its use. Today opium remains in American medicine only in the form of paregoric, camphorated tincture of opium. Many a parent has witnessed relief of their child's diarrhea by paregoric without knowing the origins of this remedy. In the past, babies born of heroin or methadone-dependent mothers, and thus themselves physically dependent, have had their withdrawal syndrome eased by paregoric.[5]

CONFESSIONS OF AN OPIUM EATER
AND OTHER PLEASURES

But, as was suggested by Homer, there is more to opium than its ability to relieve pain, fever, cough, and diarrhea. John Jones, a British physician, published a book in 1700 called *The Mysteries of Opium Reveal'd*.[6] In it he said that opium also causes "a most delicious and extraordinary refreshment of the spirits" as upon receiving "very good news or any other great cause of joy." In language bold for his day, Jones went on to say that "It has been compared not without good cause to a permanent gentle degree of that pleasure which modesty forbids the name of . . ." Modern film-makers show no such modesty. Speaking of heroin, an opioid we soon will consider, Rent-Boy, an opioid addict in the film adaptation of Irvine Welsh's novel *Trainspotting*, says this: "People think it's about misery and deprivation and death and all that shit, which is not to be ignored, but what they forget is the pleasure of it all. Otherwise we wouldn't do it. . . . Take your best orgasm, multiply by a thousand, and you're still nowhere near . . ."[7]

The smoking and eating of opium in the Orient has a long history. Indeed, so lucrative was the Chinese opium trade for the English in the 19th century that the British East India Company conducted the so-called opium wars to keep open the import of Indian opium into China.[8] In the West, the opium habit in China was generally viewed as no more than a vice among the lower levels of society, and it was little recognized that opium had become an increasingly popular drug among the working class of England as well. In any event, opium was of little interest to European intellectuals. This changed with the publication in 1821 of *The Confessions of an English Opium Eater*.[9]

The Confessor was Thomas De Quincey, who would go on to be one of England's most prolific and admired authors. De Quincey was introduced to opium at the age of 19 to relieve the pain of a toothache but soon became a regular user for reasons which he described in *The Confessions*: "For it seemed to me as if then I stood at a distance, aloof from the uproar of life; as if the tumult, the fever and the strife were suspended; a respite were granted from the secret burdens of the heart. . . . Here was the panacea for all human woes; here was the secret of happiness. . . . Thou hast the keys of paradise, O just, subtle and mighty opium."

De Quincey was not alone in his admiration for opium. Its use was a regular feature of romantic writers of the time: George Crabbe, Wilkie Collins, Francis Thompson, and John Keats in England, Charles Baudelaire in France, and Edgar Allan Poe in America were all devotees. (Some scholars have suggested that Poe was more regular in the use of opium in his writings than in person.) Samuel Taylor Coleridge wrote that his epic poem *Kubla Khan* was inspired by an opium dream. For many of these men, laudanum was the vehicle of choice, thus raising the issue of concurrent alcoholism.[10]

Despite lavishly praising the virtues of opium, De Quincey as well as medical writers of the time were aware of its more sinister aspects. In the mid-19th century, an American textbook of pharmacology noted that the use of opium was a vice, "very often pernicious in its effects," and the source of much abuse.[11] However, the author went on to say that "it does little apparent injury even through a long course of years . . . is less injurious to the individual and society than alcohol and that this evil may be corrected without great difficulty if the patient is in earnest . . ." De Quincey's view of the ease of "correction" of the opium habit, or as we would term it, opium-induced physical dependence, was less sanguine.

In *The Confessions*, De Quincey wrote that "I have struggled against this fascinating enthrallment with a religious zeal and have accomplished what I never heard attributed to any other man—have untwisted almost to its final links, the accursed chain which fettered me." We should note the inclusion of "almost" in that sentence. In fact, De Quincey soon relapsed and used opium on and off for the remaining 55 years of his life.[12] I am reminded of Mark Twain's comment that "giving up smoking is easy. I've done it many times."

MORPHINE: THE ESSENCE OF OPIUM

Pharmacologists are never pleased to deal with crude materials of unknown composition; the isolation of pure chemicals is the goal. Only in this way can precise studies be conducted and modifications of the original material be made in the search for better drugs and a clearer understanding of how they might work. It was toward that goal that a young German chemist named Friedrich Serturner began early in the 19th century to identify the chemicals in opium which might account for its remarkable properties. Summarizing his results in a classic paper published in 1817, Serturner revealed what he called "the specific narcotic element of opium."[13] Noting that it produced sleep in dogs, he named the chemical *morphine* after the god of sleep, Morpheus.

We of the 21st century, accustomed to reading about long prison sentences for the mere possession of morphine, might find Serturner's methods interesting: "To obtain a reliable assessment of morphine's action, I myself acted as a subject and asked others to do the same . . . I persuaded three people under the age of seventeen to join me in taking morphine . . ." There were no legal consequences for Serturner, as it was common for physicians and scientists of the time to experiment on themselves and on volunteers. With the isolation of morphine, one might think that opium quickly fell into obscurity, but this was hardly the case.

By the mid-1800s, the stage was set in the United States for a dramatic rise in the use of opium and its active principle, morphine. These drugs were equally attractive to physicians for whom few other effective remedies were available, to adventuresome youth as well as intellectuals influenced by De Quincey, and to the huddled masses seeking respite from their bleak lives. Often less expensive than alcohol, that other great and addictive soother of human misery, opium and morphine were freely available in every drug and grocery store without legal constraints.

OPIUM IN THE 19TH-CENTURY MARKETPLACE

Readers familiar with the Dietary Supplement Health and Education Act of 1994 are aware that sellers of vitamins, minerals, amino acids, and botanical products in the United States are free to this day to make unproven claims for the value of these materials. Our television screens are replete with these advertisements each night. The environment in the 19th century was even wilder. For one thing, as I have noted, the medical profession had few effective drugs; then as now, where no effective therapy exists, irrational therapies will thrive. Furthermore, there was little or no governmental regulation; no Food and Drug Administration existed to attempt to rein in the hucksters. Patent medicines filled the vacuum.

The active principle of *Mrs. Winslow's Soothing Syrup*, which first appeared in 1849, was morphine. For *Dr. Buckland's Scotch Oates Essence*, it was opium. The *Essence* was said to be "Nature's Nerve and Brain Food," useful for the treatment of a wide variety of ailments, including insomnia, anxiety, sciatica, paralysis, and epilepsy. Claims for *Soothing Syrup* were more modest but included was a suggestion for use in quieting irritable infants and children. Given what we know of the remarkable pharmacological properties of morphine and opium, I have no doubt that adults and children alike were often comforted by these nostrums.

A second effect, physical dependence, was certainly common, but little attention was paid. So long as patent medicines containing morphine or opium remained freely available, the withdrawal syndrome would be avoided. Years earlier the editors of the *Journal of the American Medical Association* noted the irony that of 20 "opium cures," 19 contained opium.[14] It was also said that the relative popularity of these nostrums "depends on the amount of alcohol or opium they contain." As far as the medical profession was concerned, it was stated in an authoritative textbook of pharmacology published in 1913 that "Opium . . . occupies a position of its own in therapeutics and is one of the most important and most extensively used drugs in the pharmacopeia at the present day as in the past."[15]

THE CIVIL WAR AND OUR FIRST OPIOID EPIDEMIC

Patent medicines and the unfettered marketing of these products together with widespread medical applications were certainly major factors in the prevalence of opioid use in mid-19th century America. However, it was the combination of a simple invention and the American Civil War that led to national concern about opioid physical dependence and addiction.

The shelling of Fort Sumter on April 12, 1861, marked the beginning of a war which, by its end in 1865, would claim the lives of more than 700,000 soldiers and leave countless wounded veterans. To appreciate the role that opioids would play, we must remind ourselves of the state of medical care at that time. The germ theory of disease was just that, a theory, and not accepted by most physicians. After all, some argued, if we can't see germs, how can they hurt us?

Surgeons and obstetricians would go directly from the autopsy room to the operating suite with bare hands and filthy clothing. To enter the body surgically was to invite death. To avoid infection, a battlefield wound to an arm or leg of any but the most trivial nature called for amputation. It has been estimated that there were 30,000 amputations among the Union forces alone. Opioids were freely used both at the time of operation and to deal with postoperative pain. As a result, opioid physical dependence among Civil War survivors was so prevalent that the condition came to be called "soldier's disease." This opioid epidemic, unlike that of the present day, was not accompanied by condemnation of the user or concern about the consequences. No one spoke of addiction as we define it today.

The simple invention to which I alluded was the hypodermic syringe, a hollow barrel fitted with a plunger and a beveled, hollow steel needle. With it, drugs could be delivered not only beneath the skin—hence the term *hypodermic*—but also into a muscle or other tissue or even directly into the blood via a vein. The Civil War saw the first large-scale use of the hypodermic syringe with opioids among the first drugs administered by this method. Many veterans and their relatives even learned to inject themselves.

ROUTES OF ADMINISTRATION

To appreciate the role played by the hypodermic syringe in the rise of opioid physical dependence and addiction, we need to talk a bit about routes of administration, how drugs get into our bodies. We have already been introduced to the oral route by De Quincey's "opium eating." After a drug is taken by mouth, swallowed, and absorbed into the bloodstream, it passes through the liver, where it may be altered or even inactivated. Exiting the liver, the drug reaches the general circulation for body-wide distribution. In any event, this process is relatively slow. In contrast, administration of morphine by injection into a vein allows the drug to reach its receptors in the brain very quickly and in high concentration.

Why should it matter whether a drug reaches its receptors quickly or slowly? The reason is that the rate of occupation of its receptors by a drug of dependence is a major factor in the pleasurable effects of a drug; let us call it the high. For an experienced opioid addict seeking the highest of highs, the intravenous route is nearly ideal. Unfortunately, adverse effects are also maximized. These range from sudden death to the more leisurely demise provided by bacterial and viral infections caused by dirty needles and contaminated drugs.

Before leaving the subject of routes of administration, a few words need be said about the smoking of opium. This term is a bit misleading in that, unlike the smoking of tobacco cigarettes, a process in which the tobacco is burned and nicotine vaporized in the process, opium is not burned but is merely heated to cause vaporization of the drug. The resulting fumes are then inhaled. As smokers of nicotine cigarettes and anesthesiologists are aware, inhalation is a very efficient way to introduce a drug into the body. The drug need only cross a single layer of cells in the lungs to reach the pulmonary circulation and move on to the general circulation. Indeed, this route matches that of intravenous injection in terms of speed of access to brain receptors and the high of the high without many of the hazards of intravenous administration.

HEROIN: THE DAUGHTER OF MORPHINE

With Serturner's isolation of morphine from opium, it became possible for chemists to modify the morphine structure in an attempt to find better drugs. One simple derivative, diacetylmorphine, was first marketed in Germany by F Bayer & Company in 1898, the same year that Bayer Aspirin was introduced. Diacetylmorphine was called *heroin*, a name now familiar to all.

Recommended for use in respiratory disease, heroin was said not to lead to addiction, a claim soon proven wrong. Though Consumers Union once characterized heroin as "the most hated and dreaded drug of all," this condemnation derives largely from heroin's place in the illicit market. In fact, our bodies rapidly convert heroin into morphine, and all of heroin's actions are due to morphine. Furthermore, heroin has a valued place in Great Britain for the relief of severe pain and is used in exactly the same way as is morphine in the United State. Early in the 19th century, heroin was sold to compounding pharmacies and producers of patent medicines for the treatment of pneumonia, whooping cough, and all manner of respiratory illnesses. Those in the hinterlands could consult the Sears Roebuck catalog, where heroin, together with opium, morphine, and syringes, could be purchased well into the 20th century.

Heroin hydrochloride, a water-soluble salt, is commonly taken intravenously, that is, by injection into a vein. But free base heroin, like opium, can be vaporized and the fumes inhaled, thus providing a safer route in terms of sudden death and infection. As has already been noted, drug administration by inhalation produces receptor occupation at a rate comparable to that following the intravenous route.

The smoking of heroin originated in Shanghai in the 1920s but did not reach its present form, called *chasing the dragon*, until the 1950s in Hong Kong. Free base heroin is spread on a piece of aluminum foil, heated from beneath, and the fumes inhaled via a straw. In 2010, Great Britain's Advisory Council on the Misuse of Drugs, in an effort to reduce the harm caused by intravenous use, recommended to the Secretary of State for Health that chasing the dragon be encouraged among heroin addicts by distributing foil to them.[16]

PAIN AND THE OPIOIDS

Before considering the complex issues surrounding how best to treat opioid addiction, a few more words must be said about the treatment of pain. It was William Osler, called by many the father of modern medicine, who referred to morphine as "God's own medicine."[17] No drug could have a more distinguished advocate. In 1889, he was named the first physician-in-chief of the newly founded Johns Hopkins Hospital and later would join with three others in creating the Johns Hopkins University School of Medicine. Leaving the United States at the age of 56, the Canadian-born Osler was appointed to the Regius Chair of Medicine at Oxford, named a baronet, and assumed the title of Sir William, a distinction he had long coveted. Morphine remains the standard against which all other drugs are measured for the relief of severe pain.

In chapter 1, I defined drug-induced physical dependence and contrasted it with addiction. I told you that physical dependence upon an opioid such as morphine will develop in every person treated with significant doses for an extended period of time; a terminal cancer patient provides an unambiguous example. Physical dependence is a fundamental pharmacological phenomenon, neither more nor less. Again, physical dependence is not addiction.

One of the enduring concerns about opioids in the minds of patients and their caregivers, perhaps second only to addiction, is the idea that in deadening the pain of cancer these drugs invariably cloud consciousness. Tennessee Williams provides a fictional illustration in *Cat on a Hot Tin Roof*. In the film version, Big Daddy Pollitt, the head of a prosperous Mississippi family, is suffering from terminal cancer and is in severe pain. His physician has left a supply of morphine, and his son offers an injection, saying "It will kill the pain, that's all." Big Daddy responds: "It'll kill the senses too. When you got pain at least you know you're still alive . . . I don't want to stupefy myself with that stuff."

The late Cicely Saunders would beg to differ with Big Daddy and his thoughts on the effects of opioids. First trained as a nurse during World War II and later as a physician, she had a lifelong interest in the treatment of pain and suffering particularly at the end of life. In 1967, she founded St. Christopher's Hospice in southwest London. It soon became a model for similar institutions around the world. She had this to say about drugs used at St. Christopher's.

> We find that for severe pain nothing can replace the opioids. . . . We know that nothing else will so fully ease physical and mental distress, or help the patient who feels isolated in the meaningless endurance of severe chronic pain . . . we use heroin almost exclusively. . . . Although other opioids may relieve pain just as effectively, only heroin will do so with so few side effects or leave the patient so alert and serene . . .[18]

The St. Christopher's pain-relieving mixture was composed of heroin, cocaine, gin, and an anti-nausea drug. Unfortunately, heroin is not available for medical use in the United States. Nonetheless, judicious use of opioids can be expected to provide very significant relief of pain while leaving the patient, in Dame Cicely's words, "alert and serene." (Cicely Saunders died at St. Christopher's of breast cancer at age 87.)

In 1941, the American Medical Association published a consensus paper that was intended to help "solve the problem of drug addiction." The article was entitled *Medication in the Control of Pain in Terminal Cancer*.[19] It said this: "The use of narcotic drugs in terminal cancer is to be condemned if it can possibly be avoided. . . . Morphine use is an unpleasant experience to the majority of human subjects because of undesirable side-effects. Dominant in the list of these unfortunate effects is addiction." Fortunately, the work of physicians such as Dame Cicely Saunders and others in the hospice movement exposed the myth of this position and led to a consensus in the 21st century that opioids can play a vital role in easing the departure of the terminally ill from this life. In contrast, the proper role of opioids in making more tolerable the pain of nonterminal conditions remains a matter of contention.

OPIOIDS AND THE LAW

Concurrent with the rising tide of opioid use, physical dependence, and addiction in the United States in the mid- to late 18th century, there arose an anti-opioid movement. The proponents of the movement were a mixed group. Members of the pharmacy and medical professions were not so much opposed to the sale of opioids as they were to the fact that the professions did not control this lucrative market. Prohibitionists' simply believed that all drug use is evil. There was an anti-immigrant element as well.

The western end of the transcontinental railroad was begun in Sacramento in 1863 under the guidance of the Central Pacific Railroad. Much of the prodigious amount of manual labor the project required was performed by Chinese men recruited in California and supplemented by emigrants from mainland China. Opium smoking was not uncommon among these workers, and this practice was a major factor in the passage of the Chinese Exclusion Act of 1882, which prohibited all immigration of Chinese workers.[20] The act, the first to ban a specific ethnic group, remained in effect until 1943.

Arguments by California labor unions in support of the Chinese Exclusion Act may sound familiar to those acquainted with the 2016 presidential campaigns in the United States with their extended discussion of Mexican emigrants and drugs. The Chinese were said to have alien habits, manners, and customs, including frequent drug use. Perhaps most important, the Chinese were said to reduce the living standards of "white workers."

The first two decades of the 20th century saw the passage of a number of laws related to opioids. The first of these, in 1909, prohibited the importation of opium, morphine, and heroin for other than "medicinal purposes." By 1917, these laws had been interpreted so as to prevent physicians from prescribing opioids to a physically dependent person and, more ominously, to make criminals of all those who possessed opioids for personal use. But what was to be done with these newly created criminals?

Public Law No. 672 was approved by the 70th Congress on January 19, 1929. It authorized the establishment of "two United States narcotic farms for the confinement and treatment of persons addicted to the use of habit-forming narcotic drugs who have been convicted of offenses against the United States . . ." One such offense against the United States was of course mere possession of a narcotic drug and, as had been legislated by the 67th Congress, ". . . possession shall be deemed sufficient evidence to authorize conviction . . ." The law defined an addict as "any person who habitually uses any habit-forming narcotic drug . . . so as to endanger *the public morals* (my emphasis), health, safety, or welfare . . ." The narcotic farms were to be located in Fort Worth, Texas, and Lexington, Kentucky. The stage had been set for the federal government to treat opioid addiction and to develop effective therapies.

TREATMENT: THE FARMS OF FORT WORTH AND LEXINGTON

Six years after passage of Public Law 672, the United States Narcotic Farm was opened in Kentucky.[21] The Farm was aptly named, for it sat on 1,200 acres in the heart of the Bluegrass a few miles outside Lexington. The Farm had both cattle and a dairy herd. Some called it a prison-like hospital, others a hospital-like prison. A year after opening, the Farm was officially renamed the U.S. Public Health Service Hospital. The Lexington hospital together with its sister institution which opened in Fort Worth 3 years later became the only resources in the United States for treatment of narcotic addiction. They also became centers for research using their prison population as subjects.

At the time of its opening, Lawrence C. Kolb, Sr., MD, was named chief medical officer of the Farm. Some years earlier he had written this about addicts: "The psychopath, the inebriate, the psychoneurotic, and the temperamental individuals who fall easy prey to narcotics have this in common: they are struggling with a sense of inadequacy, imagined or real or with unconscious psychological strivings that narcotics temporarily remove; and the open makeup that so many of them show is not a normal expression of men at ease with the world, but a mechanism of inferiors who are striving to appear like normal men."[22] While acknowledging the existence of a "small group of normal individuals accidentally addicted," Kolb believed that the majority of opioid addicts could be classified in the categories of "psychoneurosis, psychopathic personality, and psychosis."

The persistence of the views held by Dr. Kolb regarding addicts is witnessed by a statement made by William R. Martin, MD, 42 years after the Narcotic Farm opened: "The primary defect in the addict psychopath is that he is basically a hypophoric individual with increased needs and wants."[23] The research branch of the Lexington hospital had been renamed the Addiction Research Center (ARC) in 1948. Dr. Martin served for 13 years as the director of the ARC.

Beliefs regarding opioid addiction held by Dr. Kolb and his successors at the Lexington hospital and the ARC would shape our nation's approach to the treatment of opioid addiction until well into the 1960s. In the meantime, valuable research was conducted. Physicians and scientists at the ARC explored in a rigorous fashion in their prisoner-subjects the induction of physical dependence on morphine, methadone, and heroin as well as the features of the withdrawal syndrome for each. In addition, a number of drugs were evaluated for potential value in treating addiction. (Most research involving prisoners is now considered unethical and is generally no longer permitted.)

Treatment programs developed and implemented in the Fort Worth and Lexington hospitals evolved over the years. The guiding principle was that to achieve a permanent cure, the patient must be relieved of his emotional difficulties or taught to adjust to them without resort to narcotics. Every effort was made to maintain a drug-free environment.

A number of drugs were tested in an attempt to find a pharmacological magic bullet, but it was soon recognized that expectation of a purely medical solution to addiction was unrealistic. For this reason, trials were conducted of many modalities of treatment. Among these were psychotherapy, vocational training and work in the shops and on the farm, transcendental meditation, and group therapy, where addicts confronted each other with their evasions and denials surrounding addiction. A period of treatment of 4–6 months was thought necessary, but it was also concluded that the treatment during confinement could only start the healing process, which must be completed in the community if lifelong immunity to opioids was to be accomplished.

Unfortunately, follow-up studies revealed that at least 90% of patients resumed use of opioids within 5 years of discharge. By the criterion of enduring cure, the hospitals were a failure. By 1974, both were closed. This, I believe, is less an indictment of the hospitals and their staff than a reflection of the intractable nature of opioid addiction. Nonetheless, elements of the knowledge gained at the Public Service Hospitals with their addict-patients are to be found in every treatment program of the 21st century.

DETOXIFICATION VERSUS MEDICATION-ASSISTED THERAPY

Two of the issues addressed at the Lexington and Fort Worth hospitals were detoxification and opioid maintenance. Entering addicts still physically dependent received gradually reduced doses of morphine or codeine over a period of 14 days. In this way, signs and symptoms of the withdrawal syndrome are minimized. Addicts were then said to be "detoxified," that is, drug-free, and ready to get on with treatment.

An opioid antagonist is a drug that occupies the same receptors as does morphine or heroin but which, upon occupation of those receptors, produces no direct effect. If I am drug-free, I will be unaware that an antagonist has been given. However, in a person physically dependent on morphine, the antagonist, by blocking access of morphine to its receptors, will trigger an immediate and very severe withdrawal syndrome. With the use of an antagonist, all of these signs and symptoms appear immediately. Just as the opioid high is maximized with rapid occupation of it receptors, the severity of the withdrawal, what might be called the opioid low, is especially severe when the opioid receptors are blocked with an antagonist. What follows is how William Martin, director of the Addiction Research Center, described the natural course of the withdrawal syndrome, that is, without the use of an antagonist.

In a subject addicted to morphine, the initial abstinence symptoms emerge 6 to 12 hours after the last dose and consist of an awareness of the impending illness and feelings of restlessness, tiredness, and weakness. After 12 hours, certain signs of abstinence such as yawning, lacrimation, rhinorrhea, and perspiration emerge, as well as chills and the patient may enter into a fitful sleep called "yen sleep." After 24 hours, the patient becomes increasingly restless, twitching of various muscle groups appear, and the patient complains of neck and leg pains and has hot and cold flashes as well chills, fever, increase in both rate and depth of breathing, increased heart rate, and dilation of previously constricted pupils. By 48 hours the abstinence syndrome has neared its peak, and the patient is nauseated, retches, vomits, has diarrhea, eats and drinks very little, and loses weight rapidly. The patient may lie in a fetal position, twitching and turning and covering himself with blankets even in hot weather. After 72 hours, the syndrome begins to subside slowly . . . protracted abstinence may persist for 4–6 months . . .[24]

Three possible uses of opioid antagonists were envisioned at the Addiction Research Center in the late 1960s. The drugs studied were naloxone (Narcan) and naltrexone (Vivitrol). Of the potential uses, only one remains universally accepted today. This is reversal of the potentially lethal effects of an opioid overdose with naloxone. The drug is now being distributed to police, first responders, and addicts and their families. Many lives have been saved.

A second possibility for use of antagonists was acceleration of the onset of the withdrawal syndrome in the hope that this would somehow hasten the process of recovery. Today that approach is employed in a procedure called anesthesia-assisted rapid opioid detoxification (AAROD), in which an

antagonist is given under general anesthesia. AAROD is now regarded as
not only dangerous but also ineffective as a component of a treatment program.[25] In 2012, following two deaths in a New York City clinic, the New York
State Department of Health recommended avoidance of the procedure.
A sign of the state of regulation of the addiction treatment industry is that,
despite the advice of the New York State Department of Health and a similar condemnation by the American Society of Addiction Medicine, AAROD
is still advertised and performed in a number of clinics in the United States.

I mentioned earlier that the two major factors that maintain the use of
an opioid in an addictive fashion are the pleasurable consequences of the
drug, what behaviorists would call the reinforcing effects, and avoidance
of the withdrawal syndrome. If the pleasurable actions of the drug were to
be blocked with an antagonist, we would remove the first of these factors
and, it was hypothesized, we would have an effective treatment for addiction. That hope was only partially realized. Some addicts, having become
drug-free, find that a long-acting antagonist such as naltrexone helps them
to continue that state; heroin can no longer bring them pleasure. While attractive in theory, many addicts reject the treatment. The probable reason
is that, just as many discontinue methadone maintenance for lack of a high,
the lure of the pleasurable effects promised by the opioid is too great and
relapse occurs. It is now recognized that alternative reinforcers are needed.
Treatment programs hope to provide these alternatives.

Avoidance of the opioid withdrawal syndrome is a simple matter: Continue
the use of the opioid. Despite the tightening of controls over opioids in the
early part of the 20th century, beginning in 1919 more than 40 clinics were
established to do just that: provide morphine to addicts on a steady basis.
However, based largely on the view of the American Medical Association
that such maintenance of an opioid addict is unethical, all such clinics were
closed by the end of 1923 by the Secretary of the Treasury. The result was
that many addicts turned to illegal sources, were arrested, convicted, and
confined to federal prisons. Ironically, this dramatic increase in the con-
vict population was a prime motivating factor in the establishment of the
Narcotic Farms in Fort Worth and Lexington, where the scientific foun-
dation was laid for today's now common practice of providing opioids to
addicts as a part of an overall treatment program.

A DISEASE OR A MORAL FAILING?

In 2016, a respected physician who treats opioid addicts told me that his
patients are otherwise normal people who have inadvertently become

addicted to an opioid. Furthermore, he expressed the belief that that most addicts fit that description. Earlier I told you of the thoughts of Lawrence Kolb, the founding medical director of the Lexington Narcotic Farm.

While Dr. Kolb believed that there might be a "small group of normal individuals accidentally addicted," the majority of addicts suffered from "psychoneurosis, psychopathic personality, or psychosis," clearly not "normal people." Psychiatrists have adopted opioid addiction as a mental disorder. The most recent edition of the *Diagnostic and Statistical Manual of Mental Disorders*, published by the American Psychiatric Association, provides diagnostic criteria for opioid use disorder, which includes all of the elements of the definition of addiction we saw in the last chapter: a behavioral state of compulsive, uncontrollable drug craving and seeking which brings harm to the individual.[26]

Is opioid addiction a primary, chronic, relapsing neurobiological disease with a generally unfavorable outcome, a psychiatric disorder, or simply an absence of willpower, a moral failing, a bad habit taken to extreme? Is the addict a normal individual accidentally addicted, perhaps by a physician's well-intended opioid prescription, or a psychopath as described by Drs. Kolb and Martin?

I will not attempt to reconcile these differing views of the addict and addiction. Instead, I suggest to you that there is no "universal addict." I will instead offer my belief that the roots of addiction are multiple and often intertwined. These roots include the mental state of the individual exposed to the drugs and a multitude of other factors. Primary among the latter is a sense of hopelessness stemming from pain, suffering, a lack of stable personal relationships, poverty, or joblessness. Sigmund Freud said that we all need *Lieben und Arbeiten*, love and work, in our lives. For many, their absence may be filled by De Quincey's "panacea for all human woes."

Regardless of how we define the opioid addict, the vast majority will require treatment if their addiction is to be overcome. It is to that treatment that we now will turn.

DOLE AND NYSWANDER: OPIOID REPLACEMENT THERAPY

I have noted that, in the 1920s, clinics were opened to provide morphine to maintain opioid dependence and avoid the withdrawal syndrome. But, based on a Supreme Court ruling that it was illegal for doctors to prescribe opioids for the purposes of maintaining an addiction and the opposition to opioid maintenance by the American Medical Association, these clinics soon were closed. It was not until 1955 that the New York Academy of Medicine proposed the re-establishment of clinics and it was not until 1964 that Vincent Dole and Marie Nyswander, a wife-husband team of physician-scientists at Rockefeller University, began to treat a small number of heroin addicts with a single daily oral dose of methadone.

In 1965, Drs. Dole and Nyswander published a paper in the *Journal of the American Medical Association* entitled "A Medical Treatment for Diacetylmorphine (Heroin) Addiction: A Clinical Trial with Methadone Hydrochloride.[27] New York City at that time was said to be home to 50% of all the heroin addicts in the country. As heroin addicts, all were regarded as criminals. In a remarkable departure from existing ideas about heroin addiction, Dole and Nyswander proposed that the addicts suffered from a chronic disease which could be corrected by an opioid; in effect, the addicts had been self-medicating.

The investigators chose methadone as a substitute drug based upon what had been learned years earlier from the prisoners at Lexington's narcotic hospital. While methadone has all of the properties of heroin, it is longer acting, stable blood levels can be achieved when taken by mouth, and normal functioning maintained. This is in contrast with heroin, which, even with multiple daily injections, produces alternating highs and lows, thus making heroin, in their view, unsuitable for maintenance therapy. Dole and Nyswander reported that addicts on stabilized doses of methadone "lost their craving for narcotics and appeared functionally normal in all respects." In addition, if the maintenance dose of methadone was sufficiently high, a generalized opioid tolerance would deny an addict any pleasure from his usual dose of street heroin. Thus began what today is called opioid replacement therapy (ORT), which in turn is often a component of medication-assisted treatment (MAT).

In the more than half century since the birth of ORT, only one addition has been made. That was the approval in 2002 of buprenorphine. Like methadone, buprenorphine is an opioid with all the properties of an opioid; it is able to relieve pain, induce physical dependence, produce euphoria, and cause death in overdose. Its therapeutic virtue is that it is an opioid partial agonist, a drug which acts on opioid receptors but which produces maximal effects less than full agonists such as heroin. Because of this "ceiling effect," it is less likely to suppress breathing and kill in overdose—think of it as Methadone Lite. A practical consideration for addicts and those who would treat them is that, unlike methadone maintenance, which is conducted out of strictly controlled clinics, buprenorphine can be prescribed in an office setting by any physician who completes an 8-hour certification program. In recent years, several long-acting formulations of buprenorphine have been approved; one of these is a depot preparation that lasts for 6 months. In 2019, a form administered by monthly injection [Sublocade] was approved for use in the United States.

Today thousands of addicts are maintained on buprenorphine or methadone for extended periods of time while measures are taken to address the underlying roots of their addiction. But the controversy that surrounded Dole and Nyswander in the 1960s did not end. When a proposal was made in 1998 to expand the methadone programs in New York City, its then mayor Rudolph Guiliani expressed the view that this would only make more people "addicted to methadone which is perhaps a worse addiction."[28] Today that view is shared by many who advocate abstinence-only programs. In the words of *Dawn Farm*, an addiction treatment program in Ypsilanti, Michigan, opioid replacement therapy "is neither necessary nor helpful." We will return to these issues in chapter 9.

As concern about an opioid epidemic has risen, previously rejected ideas for treatment have been reconsidered. In choosing a drug for maintenance therapy, Dole and Nyswander dismissed heroin because of its short duration of action. However, with the observation that many addicts prematurely leave methadone maintenance programs or opioid antagonist therapy, perhaps because they can no longer experience the pleasurable effects of an opioid, those advocating heroin as a maintenance drug have come forward.

In 1926, a report was presented to the British government by the Rolleston Committee, a group that had been created to provide direction on opioid use.[29] They concluded that supplying addicts with heroin for maintenance constitutes legitimate medical practice if such maintenance enabled the addict to live "a normal useful life." In what came to be called the British System, addiction was considered an illness rather than criminal behavior. The System appears to have worked well until, in the 1960s, an increase in addiction to heroin among young people was attributed to overprescribing by physicians. Tighter controls, including the identification of addicts to a governmental agency, were then instituted, but the provision of heroin to addicts has continued.

Great Britain is not alone. In Switzerland, pilot projects were begun in 1994, and heroin prescription became legal in 1998. Similar programs are now in place in the Netherlands, Denmark, and Germany.

Heroin maintenance in a modified form came to North America with the founding in 2003 of Insite, a supervised injection facility in Vancouver, British Columbia.[30] Addicts bring illicit heroin to the clinic, where sterile injection equipment and nurse supervision are provided. If desired, detoxification, counseling, and other treatment modalities are available. With the success of Insite in reducing overdose deaths and HIV/AIDS among addicts, true heroin maintenance began in Vancouver in 2005 with the founding of the Crosstown Clinic, where pure heroin for injection is provided free of charge. The Clinic has continued in operation despite legal challenges from Canada's Conservative Party, which is generally opposed to harm-reduction policies.

Whether heroin maintenance will spread across Canada, or even to the United States, remains to be seen. It is obviously a much tougher sell than is maintenance with methadone or buprenorphine. Alan Freedman reported in *The Washington Post* in September 2016 that Scott MacDonald, the physician-in-chief at the Crosstown Clinic, met resistance following a presentation in Boston. Dr. MacDonald said that "there were physicians who would not even come up and talk to me." When, in 2019, a group called Safehouse attempted to open a supervised injection site for opioids in Philadelphia, the United States Justice Department filed a suit in District Court asking that such sites be declared illegal.

THE ADDICTION TREATMENT INDUSTRY

Addiction treatment is a multi-billion-dollar industry. The National Association of Addiction Treatment Providers publishes an *Addiction Industry Directory*. The directory lists 581 "Accredited Providers." Its participants range from grim methadone maintenance facilities funded by government agencies to "luxury rehabilitation" at places such as Seasons in Malibu; the latter provides a private room at a cost of $72,500 per month; their advertisements are quick to mention that "This is a cash pay facility."

Some programs, with licensed physicians on their staff, provide opioid replacement therapy in the form of methadone or buprenorphine coupled with a variety of behavioral interventions. Others are emphatically opposed to medication-assisted therapy as just another form of addiction. In addition, the use of drugs is under the control of the medical profession and there are many who distrust organized medicine, thinking it merely a vehicle for enriching doctors and drug companies. As an alternative, these groups often employ medication-free methods, often referred to as abstinence-only programs, developed in the 1930s by Alcoholics Anonymous. So-called 12-step programs feature the admission that one's addiction is out of control, recognition of a higher power, and making amends for past errors.

Cost of treatment aside, what works? Comparison of the success rates for abstinence-only versus opioid replacement therapy is made difficult by the relapsing nature of addiction, an absence of standards for what constitutes success, and wholly inadequate regulation of the addiction treatment industry. It is the view of Richard D. Blondell, MD, director of the National Center for Physician Training in Addiction Medicine, that abstinence-only programs have a success rate of 15%–20%, but for those then entering maintenance therapy, 40%–50% will recover.

NARCO FREEDOM OR NARCO FRAUD?

Among the 581 treatment providers listed in the *Addiction Industry Directory*, there are many fine programs. However, in a report issued by the National Center on Addiction and Substance Abuse, a nonprofit organization focused on improving the treatment of addiction, it was pointed out that there are no national standards for the provision of addiction treatment. Their conclusion was that "few addicts receive anything that approximates evidence-based care."[31] Furthermore, "most of those providing addiction care are not medical professionals and are not equipped with the knowledge, skills, or credentials to provide the full range of effective treatments." Most states do not require that addiction counselors have advanced education of any kind. In the worst of these programs, outright fraud is perpetrated. Narco Freedom will serve as an example.

Founded in 1971, Narco Freedom initially provided methadone treatment to addicts in the South Bronx area of New York City. Licensed by the New York State Department of Health, its services expanded over the years to serve alcoholics, the mentally ill, and the homeless throughout the city. In October 2014, the chief executive officer of Narco Freedom and his son were indicted on charges of fraud and money laundering. These charges were expanded in March 2015 to include corruption, grand larceny, and bribery. One of Narco Freedom's tactics was to encourage prison parolees to live in "Freedom Houses" owned by the company. A condition of housing was to enter into methadone maintenance and to receive addiction counseling three to seven times per week. For each session, Narco Freedom billed Medicaid $84. For all of its activities in 2015, Narco Freedom received in excess of $40,000,000 in Medicaid funds. It has been said that the wheels of justice turn slowly; 40 years earlier, just 5 years after its founding, Narco Freedom was presented to a Senate committee to illustrate fraud among methadone maintenance programs.[32]

In his fiscal year 2017 budget, President Obama called on the US Congress to provide $1.1 billion "to expand access to treatment in communities across the country," including $920 million for improved access to medication-assisted therapy for opioid addiction. Impressive as this might appear, the amounts proposed by President Trump to fight the opioid epidemic for each of the years 2018 and 2019 exceeded $12 billion. Alas, in the absence of more stringent governmental control of addiction treatment programs, I fear that much of any increased funding will be lost to fraud by groups such as Narco Freedom.

DAVID LIVINGSTON AND ENDORPHINS

I will close this chapter with an account by Lewis Thomas of a near-death experience by David Livingstone, a Scotsman and the most famous of the 19th-century medical missionary-explorers of Africa.

> He was caught by a lion, crushed across the chest in the animal's great jaws, and saved in the instant by a lucky shot from a friend. Later, he remembered the episode in clear detail. He was so amazed by the extraordinary sense of peace, calm, and total painlessness associated with being killed that he constructed a theory that all creatures are provided with a protective physiological mechanism, switched on at the verge of death, carrying them through in a haze of tranquility.[33]

A physiological basis for Livingston's observation was provided in the 1970s by the discovery of a family of naturally occurring chemicals in the brain which have many of the properties of opioids.[34] These chemicals are now collectively called endorphins. They are the transmitters in the human body's analgesic system. Morphine and other opioids merely mimic the action of these endogenous substances but in a very powerful way. In pop psychology, release of endorphins is commonly invoked to explain the joy of sex, exercise, food, and other pleasurable human activities.

Earlier I said that if I am drug-free, I will be unaware that I have received an opioid antagonist such as naloxone. But if my own opioids, the endorphins, are always present, I would expect naloxone to precipitate a withdrawal syndrome. The fact that it does not suggests that the endogenous system envisaged by Dr. Livingston is switched on only during times of great stress, as, for example, while being "caught by a lion." In the search for nonaddictive pain relievers, many have searched for ways in which the actions of the endorphins might be enhanced, but no success has yet been achieved.

NOTES

1. Holmstedt B, Liljestrand G (1963) *Readings in Pharmacology*. London: Pergamon Press.

2. Holmstedt B, Liljestrand G (1963) *Readings in Pharmacology*. London: Pergamon Press.

3. Berridge V (1999) *Opium and the People*. London: Free Association Books.

4. Sydenham T (1676) *Medical Observations Concerning the History and Cure of Acute Diseases*. London: The Sydenham Society.

5. Bio LL, Siu A, Poon CY (2011) Update on the pharmacologic management of neonatal abstinence syndrome. *J Perinatol* 31(11):692–701.

6. Estes JW (1979) John Jones's *Mysteries of Opium Reveal'd (1701): Key to Historical Opiates*. *J Hist Med Allied Sci* 34(2):200–210.

7. Welsh I (1993) *Trainspotting*. London: Secker & Warburg.

8. Lovell J (2011) *The Opium Wars: Drugs, Dreams, and the Making of China*. London: Picador.

9. De Quincey T (1822) *Confessions of an English Opium-eater*. 1966 edition edited by A. Ward. New York: New American Library.

10. Todd J (1968) Drug addiction and artistic genius. *The Practitioner* 201:513–523.

11. Wood GB (1856) *A Treatise on Therapeutics and Pharmacology or Materia Medica*. Philadelphia: Lippincott.

12. Schiller F (1976) Thomas De Quincey's lifelong addiction. *Perspec Biol Med* Autumn: 131–141.

13. Serturner FWA (1817) Ueber das Morphium, eine neue salzfahige Grundlage, und die Mekonsaure, als Hauptbestandetheile des Opiums. *Gilbert's Ann d. Physik* (Leipzig) 25:56–89.

14. Anonymous (1888) How the opium habit is acquired. *JAMA* 313(5):1597.

15. Cushny AR (1913) *A Textbook of Pharmacology and Therapeutics*. Philadelphia: Lea & Febiger.

16. Advisory Council on the Misuse of Drugs (2010) The consideration of the use of foil to reduce the harms of injecting heroin. London: UK Home Office Publications.

17. Golden RL (2009) William Osler, urolithiasis, and God's own medicine. *Urology* 74(3):517–521.

18. Saunders C (2000) The evolution of palliative care. *Patient Educ Couns* 41(1):226–2235.

19. Lee LE (1941) Medication in the control of pain in terminal cancer. *JAMA* 116:216–219.

20. OurDocuments.gov (2018) Chinese Exclusion Act of 1882. www.ourdocuments.gov/doc.php?flash=true&doc=47

21. Martin WR, Isbell H (1978) *Drug Addiction and the U.S. Public Health Service*. DHEW Publication No. (ADM) 77–434. Washington, D.C.: U.S. Government Printing Office.

22. Martin WR, Isbell H (1978) *Drug Addiction and the U.S. Public Health Service*. DHEW Publication No. (ADM) 77–434. Washington, D.C.: U.S. Government Printing Office.

23. Martin WR, Isbell H (1978) *Drug Addiction and the U.S. Public Health Service*. DHEW Publication No. (ADM) 77–434. Washington, D.C.: U.S. Government Printing Office.

24. Martin WR (1977) *Drug Addiction I*, W. R. Martin, Ed. New York: Springer-Verlag.

25. Centers for Disease Control and Prevention (2013) Deaths and severe adverse events associated with anesthesia-assisted rapid opioid detoxification—New York City, 2012. *MMWR Morb Mortal Wkly Rep* 62(38):777–780.

26. American Psychiatric Association (2013) *Diagnostic and Statistical Manual of Mental Disorders*, 5th edition. Washington, D.C.: APA.

27. Dole VP, Nyswander M (1965) A medical treatment for diacetylmorphine (heroin) addiction: A clinical trial with methadone hydrochloride. *JAMA* 193:80–84.

28. Ciment J (1998) Clash in US over methadone treatment. *The Lancet* 252:1205.

29. Report of the Departmental Committee on Morphine and Heroin Addiction (Rolleston) (1926) London: Her Majesty's Stationary Office.

30. Insite—Supervised Injection Site (2016) http://suervisedinjection.vch.ca/

31. CASA Columbia (2012) *Addiction Medicine: Closing the Gap Between Science and Practice.* www.centeronaddiction.org/addiction-research/reports/addiction-medicine-closing-gap-between-science- and- practice

32. Special Committee on Aging (1976) *The Narco Freedom Case.* Washington, D.C.: U.S. Government Printing Office.

33. Jeal T (2013) *Livingstone: Revised and Expanded Edition.* New Haven, CT: Yale University Press.

34. Brownstein MJ (1993) A brief history of opiates, opioid peptides, and opioid receptors. *Proc Natl Acad Sci* 90:5391–5393.

CHAPTER 3

 oⱱ⦵

Marijuana

From Reefer Madness to THC Gummy Bears

No substance better exemplifies the ambivalence of Western societies toward psychoactive drugs than marijuana. In 2017, it was estimated that there were more than 22 million current users, about 6.7% of the adult population, in the United States. For those aged 18 to 25, the figure was nearly 20%.[1] In the United Kingdom, the prevalence of recreational use of marijuana among males aged 16–34 was put at 15.5%.[2] Despite its widespread acceptance, many regard marijuana as a serious drug of abuse which, if set free, will destroy the fabric of our society.[3] Others see it as one of God's gifts to humankind and regularly call for its legalization for medical use. By 2018, the United Kingdom and 40 other countries had heeded that call. In the United States, medical marijuana has been approved in 30 states and the District of Columbia with more sure to follow. Going further, recreational use is allowed in 10 of those states. Nonetheless, marijuana possession continues to be illegal under federal law in the United States, and some physicians have been threatened with loss of their licenses for advocating medical marijuana.[4] In 2015, combined state and federal laws led to more arrests for possession of small amounts of marijuana than those for all violent crimes combined.[5]

Our Love Affair with Drugs: The History, the Science, the Politics. Jerrold Winter, Oxford University Press (2020). © Jerrold Winter.
DOI: 10.1093/oso/9780190051464.001.0001

CANNABIS SATIVA

The word *marijuana* (or the alternate spelling *marihuana*) does not appear in American medical texts of the 19th century. Instead, the term *cannabis* referred to flowering tops of the female plant of *Cannabis sativa*. At that time, while millions of persons in Asia and Africa habitually indulged in cannabis as an intoxicant, cannabis was little used for that purpose in this country. In this chapter, I will use the term "cannabis" to refer to any active material derived from *Cannabis sativa* and *Cannabis indica*, the two species—some say subspecies—of the plant.

Today's controversies surrounding "medical marijuana" often ignore its long history in European and American medicine. Beginning in 1850, *Cannabis indica* and several extracts of the plant were listed in *The United States Pharmacopeia*, an official compilation of medically useful drugs. They were not removed from the publication until 1942. Writing in 1890 in *The Lancet*, John Russell Reynolds, physician to Queen Victoria's household, expressed the view that cannabis is "one of the most valuable medicines we possess."[6] Sir John recommended cannabis for the treatment of a variety of ailments, including migraine, depression, asthma, and epilepsy. We shall return later to the 21st-century controversies surrounding the use of chemicals derived from cannabis in therapy for epilepsy and for chronic pain.

TETRAHYDROCANNABINOL

Although cannabis has been used by humans for thousands of years, its story is easier told if we first jump ahead to its modern history, which comprises four chapters. The first begins in 1945 when Alexander Todd, professor of chemistry at the University of Cambridge, obtained 5 tons of marijuana which had been seized from smugglers by the Egyptian government.[7] From this ample supply, Professor Todd distilled what came to be called "red oil." A mere 70 milligrams (seventeen-hundredths of an ounce) of the oil produced an intoxication lasting several hours. (Sir Alexander went on to win the Nobel Prize in Chemistry for work unrelated to marijuana.)

The second chapter in the modern history of cannabis opened in 1964. It was in that year that Raphael Mechoulam of Hebrew University in Jerusalem isolated the primary pharmacologically active principle of marijuana.[8] Its name is (-)-delta-9-tetrahydrocannabinol; I will refer to it as THC. It is now recognized that cannabis contains 100 or more distinct chemicals, which we will refer to as cannabinoids, but THC remains of central importance. Forms of cannabis may differ markedly in pharmacological activity, but these are usually explicable on the basis of their THC content. Although the THC content of marijuana cigarettes has tended to increase over the past several decades, it rarely exceeds 10%, whereas hashish, the concentrated resin from marijuana, could come in at 65% THC.

It cannot be argued that Mechoulam's identification of THC as the drug responsible for the major effects of cannabis signaled an age of enlightenment in our legal dealings with the plant. What the discovery of THC most certainly accomplished was to permit scientific investigation of the pharmacological properties of cannabis in all its forms. From the largely imagined high of farm boys smoking weeds to drug-driven flights from reality by big-city connoisseurs of hashish, the spectrum of the effects of cannabis could now be rationalized in terms of THC content.

THE ENDOCANNABINOID SYSTEMS

In the previous chapter on opioids, we saw how the discovery of the opioid receptor led to the identification of substances found in our brains which mimic the effects of opioids. These endogenous ligands were given the name *endorphins*. In a similar manner, the third and fourth chapters of our modern history of marijuana begin with the discovery of a cannabinoid receptor. In 1988, the American pharmacologists William Devane, Allyn Howlett, and their coworkers characterized a cannabinoid receptor in rat brain.[9] Devane would later join Mechoulam in Israel, and by 1992 they and their associates had isolated a chemical which is present in all of our brains and acts on cannabinoid receptors.[10] This endogenous ligand, a derivative of arachidonic acid, was given the name *anandamide* from the Sanskrit word for "bliss." With these discoveries, THC joined the opioids in having a physiological system upon which to act and natural mediators to mimic.[11]

A year following the discovery of anandamide, a second cannabinoid receptor was identified.[12] Unlike the receptor for THC, which is located primarily within the brain, this second receptor is mostly found in the periphery, that is, outside of the central nervous system, on cells of the immune system in organs such as the spleen, tonsils, and thymus. To distinguish the two receptors, that occupied by THC is designated CB_1, while the second is called CB_2. The chemical components of cannabis act to varying degrees on the CB_1 and CB_2 receptors. We will occupy ourselves with just two: THC acting on CB_1 to produce marijuana's behavioral effects and cannabidiol (CBD, originally identified in 1940), which occupies the CB_2 receptor and is devoid of psychoactivity. But THC and CBD are pharmacologically promiscuous in that each acts both on CB_1 and on CB_2 receptors.

Later we will return to the combination of THC and CBD in our discussion of the treatment of childhood epilepsy.

TEN THOUSAND YEARS OF CANNABIS

The beginning of the ancient era of cannabis is uncertain, but two properties made the plant attractive to humans. The first has to do with the effects of THC on the body, especially the brain, the second, with the nature of the stalk. When cannabis is cut down and allowed to rot, one is left with long, tough fibers which can be woven into rope and coarse cloth. Another name for *Cannabis sativa* is Indian hemp. Surely hemp and its products were some of the earliest articles of human commerce.

Exactly when or where the properties of cannabis as an intoxicant were first recognized is not known. Richard Evans Schultes and Albert Hofmann suggest the Altai Mountains of Central Asia perhaps 10,000 years ago.[13] We do know that by the time of Christ, cannabis was used as a source of fiber and as an intoxicant throughout vast areas of China, India, Southeast Asia, and Africa. As is true of many other psychoactive plants, cannabis often became a part of local religious practices, witchcraft, magic, and medicine.

Although cannabis was known in Europe by about the 2nd century B.C., little attention was paid it until just a few hundred years ago; Europeans tended to regard intoxication with cannabis as but another barbarism of those from the East. The land bridge from Asia to the New World disappeared before cannabis could enter, so the Americas had to wait until the 16th century for African slaves or their European masters to introduce the plant.

In the American colonies, hemp was commonly grown as a source of fiber and, although the record is fragmentary, was probably known for its intoxicating properties as well. Benjamin Franklin, writing in his *Pennsylvania Gazette* in 1728, describes the making of rope from the common hemp plant. After drying the material, the worker is told to burn off the leaves. But, Franklin cautions, " . . . do not stand in the smoke for it makes the head feel funny."[14] Among the early hemp farmers was George Washington of Mount Vernon, Virginia.

THE DOSE–RESPONSE RELATIONSHIP FOR THC

The vast majority of drugs produce a spectrum of effects which is related in an orderly fashion to the amount of drug taken; pharmacologists speak of a "dose–response relationship." (An exception to this general principle occurs when allergic or immunologic responses occur.) Before we consider the legal and social and, some would say, moral issues which surround cannabis, we need to examine the dose–response relationship for THC. Given the fact that millions of Americans have experienced the effects of low doses of marijuana, I am perhaps carrying coals to Newcastle in providing the following description. Most commonly the drug produces a dreamy, relaxed state in which thinking seems, on the one hand, free and unbounded and, on the other, disrupted and disjointed. The senses of vision and hearing are enhanced while time seems to move more slowly. All of these low-dose effects of THC are profoundly influenced by the circumstances in which the drug is used, the setting, and by the initial state of mind of the user, the set. In a group setting some will giggle and laugh, while others withdraw quietly. Friends may become friendlier and lovers more loving. Experience with the drug is important: First-time users are often unimpressed, while a devotee reliably obtains the desired results.

Until recently, the effects of higher doses of THC were unfamiliar to most Americans for the simple reason that most marijuana was too dilute a source of the drug. To experience the far end of the dose–response relationship one needs a more potent form of cannabis, a more concentrated source of THC. In the laboratory one can use THC itself, but for centuries hashish, the resin scraped from the leaves of cannabis, served quite nicely.

I need not struggle with a description of the effects of hashish, that is, a high dose of THC, because many others, far more eloquent than I, have left us their accounts of the experience. Theophile Gautier, a French poet of the 19th century, wrote as follows:

> It seemed that my body was dissolving and becoming transparent. I could clearly see in my chest the hashish I had eaten, in the form of an emerald glowing with a million sparkles. My eyelashes grew to infinity and like golden threads wound around little ivory spindles that spun by themselves with dazzling speed. About me were rivers, nay torrents of gems of all colors, with endlessly changing floral patterns that I can only compare with kaleidoscopic patterns. I still saw my comrades in certain situations but distorted, half men, half plants, with the pensive air of ibises standing on one leg and flapping their wings. They were so strange that I was convulsed with laughter in my corner. To join the fun, I began tossing my cushions in the air, catching them and throwing them with the dexterity of an Indian juggler. One of the guests addressed me in Italian, which hashish, in its omnipotence, changed into Spanish. The questions and answers were almost reasonable and touched upon such important subjects as literature and the theater. . . .What is different about hashish intoxication is that it is not

continuous; it takes you and it leaves you; you rise to heaven and you fall back to earth without transition. As with insanity, there are lucid moments . . . [15]

With the identification of THC as the major psychoactive component of cannabis, laboratory studies provided confirmation of Gautier's observations. Although the descriptions were considerably more prosaic, they left no doubt that THC is hallucinogenic at high doses.[1617]

The idea that hashish might produce a state akin to insanity was particularly attractive to Jacques-Joseph Moreau, a French psychiatrist and friend of Gautier. In 1845, Moreau published a book titled *Hashish and Mental Illness*.[18] In it, he described the effects of hashish which he had observed in others during his travels in the Orient, in himself, and upon a group which Gautier named *Le Club des Hachichins*, a mix of Parisian artists, writers, scientists, and generic bon vivants with a common interest in states of intoxication.

As we might expect from the title of his book, Moreau thought that hashish produced a state much like insanity. But he thought as well that hashish could be useful as a treatment for mental illness and he related some of the favorable effects he had seen in his depressed patients. Gautier made the suggestion to Moreau that the drug might have value in "expanding" the minds of the mentally retarded. All of this, of course, has a familiar ring to observers of the drug scene since the 1960s. Virtually every psychoactive drug, certainly marijuana, has been claimed by some to cause mental illness while others propose the use of such drugs as aids to mental health and stability.

MARIJUANA AND THE LAW

The attitude of the American public toward marijuana in the early years of the 20th century was shaped in large measure by society's perception of those who used the drug. So long as marijuana use was confined to migrant farm workers from Mexico and jazz musicians and a few members of the upper and lower classes in places like New Orleans and New York City, the great mass of Americans paid it little attention. From time to time the public would be titillated by a story of sex, murder, or mayhem purportedly committed while intoxicated by the plant. A few people went to prison for 10 or 20 years or longer for possession, but they were nearly always regarded as social deviants of one kind or another who would be locked up for something else if it were not for marijuana. The vast majority of Americans had no direct experience with the plant; it was simply irrelevant.

Earlier I mentioned the place of cannabis in American medicine of that time; it had accepted uses, but there was no great enthusiasm as to its efficacy. But one aspect of the early medical accounts of the effects of cannabis would have far-reaching effects on the laws which were to come. Albert Cushny's *The Action of Drugs in Health and Disease*, a text published in 1913 and intended for use by physicians and other health professionals, is typical: "The effects of Cannabis indica are chiefly due to changes in the brain where it produces a mixture of depression and stimulation *similar to that seen under morphine* (my emphasis)."[19]

HARRY ANSLINGER AND REEFER MADNESS

Until 1932, the federal government paid little attention to marijuana. But on the first day of that year, Harry Jacob Anslinger became commissioner of the Federal Bureau of Narcotics, an organization created 2 years earlier. During his quarter-century reign, Anslinger's passionate desire to eliminate the use of what he called "this lethal weed" never cooled. Largely through his efforts, anti-marijuana laws were passed in each of the United States and the Marihuana Tax Act of 1937 required the registration of all those who possessed the drug.[20] A year later, the Uniform Narcotic Drug Act defined narcotic drugs as "coca leaves, opium, cannabis and every substance not chemically distinguishable from them"; cannabis and opium had been legally linked.[21]

Unfortunately, such notions about similarities between opium and cannabis persisted long after it became clear that their properties are distinctly different. As we saw in the preceding chapter, opium and drugs such as morphine, heroin, and oxycodone can lead to highly significant physical dependence, whereas cannabis does not; opioids readily kill in overdose, whereas cannabis does not; the addictive potential of opioids is orders of magnitude greater than that of cannabis; the pharmacological receptors upon which opioids act are distinctly different than those which mediate the effects of THC and the cannabinoids. These errors of pharmacological fact would lead to enormous difficulties in writing sensible laws and in other efforts designed to control the use of cannabis.

A book by Harry Anslinger and William Tompkins, the United States Attorney for the State of New Jersey, was titled *The Traffic in Narcotics*.[22] In it, we are told the following about cannabis:

> Whereas the opioids can be a blessing when properly used, marijuana has no therapeutic value, and its use is therefore always an abuse and a vice. . . . While

opium can be a blessing or a curse depending on its use, marijuana is only and always a scourge which undermines its victims and degrades them mentally, morally, and physically. . . . In the earliest stages of intoxication, the will power is destroyed and inhibitions and restraints are released; the moral barricades are broken down and often debauchery and sexuality results. When mental instability is inherent, the behavior is generally violent. An egotist will enjoy delusions of grandeur, the timid individual will suffer anxiety, and the aggressive one often will resort to acts of violence and crime. Dormant tendencies are released and while the subject may know what is happening, he has become powerless to prevent it. Constant use produces an incapacity for work and a disorientation of purpose. The drug has a corroding effect on the body and on the mind, weakening the entire physical system and often leading to insanity after prolonged use.

To anyone wishing a visual representation of the Anslinger school of information on marijuana, I recommend *Reefer Madness,* a film made in 1936 but still available today. Eighty years after its creation, I watched it once again on a Netflix DVD. Teenage smokers of marijuana who view *Reefer Madness* will of course reject its contents as camp, distorted and dishonest. As one of them put it: "All of my friends smoke pot and none of them are crazy." Unfortunately, teens may reject as distorted and dishonest all the truths there are to be told about cannabis and nicotine and heroin and alcohol and cocaine and LSD and all the rest of the drugs which, to a greater or lesser extent, are available to them.

A SPECTACULAR RESURGENCE

Somewhere sometime in the early 1960s, cannabis began its rise. One wise commentator called it a "spectacular resurgence." Perhaps first on college campuses but soon in every corner of our society pot smoking became fashionable. By the end of the decade, surveys indicated that nearly half of all young adults had sampled the drug and perhaps 10 million were regular users. Law enforcement agencies were not idle: In the period between 1965 and 1970, arrests under state marijuana laws increased 10-fold; the courts and the jails were swamped. Parents across the country were suddenly faced with the prospect of their children being imprisoned as felons. Lawyers rejoiced; I recall talking with a young attorney in 1968 who had all the business he could handle at $500 per marijuana arrest.

It soon became clear that if the laws against marijuana were rigorously applied, a significant fraction of our otherwise law-abiding citizens would become criminals. An intolerable situation; you cannot jail doctors and bankers and dentists and business leaders, not to mention their sons and daughters and perhaps even their legal counselors. Across the country there was a turning away from the marijuana laws; sheriffs could no longer make the front page of the Sunday paper simply by raiding a Saturday night pot party at the local college.

NATIONAL COMMISSIONS WEIGH IN

On the federal level, the Comprehensive Drug Abuse Prevention and Control Act of 1970 was passed.[23] Long and detailed, two features of the Act stand out. The first of these was the establishment of five Schedules of controlled substances. A drug placed in Schedule I has (a) a high potential for abuse, (b) no accepted medical use in the United States, and (c) a lack of accepted safety for use of the drug under medical supervision. Among the many Schedule I drugs explicitly listed in the Act were opioids such as heroin, hallucinogens including LSD, and marijuana. However, for the first time, a distinction was made between opioids and marijuana in terms of penalties attached to their possession, sale, or use. For opioids, the penalty was not more than 15 years' imprisonment but for marijuana just 5 years. The Act also called for the creation of a commission that would recommend drug abuse policy to the President and to the Congress of the United States.

The National Commission on Marijuana and Drug Abuse submitted its report on March 22, 1972. It still makes interesting reading. After a careful review of the then-existent data, the Commission considered three possibilities: total prohibition, partial prohibition, and legalization. What follows is taken from the Commission's report *Marijuana: A Signal of Misunderstanding*.[24]

> The total prohibition scheme was rejected primarily because no sufficiently compelling social reason, predicated on existing knowledge, justifies intrusion into the private lives of individuals who use marijuana. The Commission is of the unanimous opinion that marijuana use is not such a grave problem that individuals who smoke marijuana, and possess it for that purpose, should be subject to criminal procedures. . . . Considering the range of social concerns in contemporary America, marijuana does not, in our considered judgement, rank very high. We would deemphasize marijuana as a problem.

The National Commission on Marijuana and Drug Abuse was not, we must remind ourselves, a radical group. Its members had been appointed by President Richard M. Nixon, and they were chaired by Raymond Shafer, a former Republican governor of Pennsylvania. Furthermore, their findings and recommendations differed little from those of similarly prestigious and conservative groups in England and in Canada. In the United States, a study commissioned by New York City Mayor Fiorello La Guardia and published in 1944,[25] refuted many of the claims regarding marijuana made by Harry Anslinger, who labeled the report as being unscientific.

Within a few years after the Commission's findings, several states, beginning with Oregon in 1973, decriminalized the possession for personal use of small amounts of marijuana. Efforts to remove criminal penalties were led by organizations such as the National Organization for the Reform of Marijuana Laws (NORML). On the other hand, many Americans remained convinced of marijuana's power to do harm to those who use it. They continued to seize upon every suggestion of cannabis's toxicity; distraught parents invoked marijuana as the reason for their children's lack of interest in church or school. As a result, there was constant pressure to restudy marijuana.

A decade following *Marijuana: A Signal of Misunderstanding*, the results of a study commissioned by the National Institute on Drug Abuse were published with the title *An Analysis of Marijuana Policy*.[26] It was acknowledged that "marijuana is not a harmless drug (and that) prolonged or excessive use may cause serious harmful biological and social effects in many users." The report expressed particular concern about "its potential effects on the psychological development of adolescents." However, it was also found that there had been no change in the overall balance between the costs and benefits of total prohibition; criminalization of users was in their view an inappropriate response to the known and suspected hazards of marijuana use. They concluded, just as had the Schafer committee a decade earlier, "that a policy of partial prohibition is clearly preferable to a policy of complete prohibition of supply and use."

An Analysis of Marijuana Policy received less than a warm welcome in some circles. Critics of the committee's recommendations pointed out that marijuana was mentioned in 2.3% of the reports from hospital emergency rooms monitored by the Drug Abuse Warning Network in 1980; others noted that aspirin appeared in 3.3%. And so it went and so it goes.

In 1972, the National Commission on Marijuana and Drug Abuse expressed their "unanimous opinion that marijuana use is not such a grave problem that individuals who smoke marijuana, and possess it for that purpose, should be subject to criminal procedures." In 2011, 39 years later, Lee Carroll Brooker of Dothan, Alabama, was sentenced to life imprisonment without the possibility of parole for the crime of growing marijuana plants.[27] Mr. Brooker, a disabled veteran, used the marijuana to treat his chronic pain. In 2016, Jeffrey Beauregard Sessions, the senior senator from Mr. Brooker's state of Alabama, told a U.S. Senate committee that "Good people don't smoke marijuana."[28] The following year, Mr. Sessions, having been appointed Attorney General of the United States, told a group of police chiefs that marijuana is "nearly as dangerous as heroin."[29]

MEDICAL MARIJUANA AND *CATCH-22*

Joseph Heller flew 60 missions as a B-25 bombardier with the U.S. Army Air Force in the European theater during World War II. Based on that experience, he wrote a novel in which Captain John Yossarian, like Heller, a bombardier, encounters an obscure Air Force regulation, *Catch-22*, which gives title to the book.[30] As explained by the squadron doctor, if you are crazy, you can't be obliged to continue flying combat missions; you need only ask to be relieved. The catch is that only a sane person would make the request to be relieved; this proves that you are not crazy, so you must continue to fly.

The catch-22 for marijuana is derived from the Comprehensive Drug Abuse Prevention and Control Act of 1970.[31] In it, marijuana was placed in Schedule I, making it illegal for clinical study. Thus, marijuana cannot be moved from Schedule I to Schedule II unless there is clinical evidence of medical benefit, but that evidence cannot be obtained so long as it remains in Schedule I. Progress in establishing both the medical efficacy and the possible hazards of cannabis use has been very significantly slowed by this legal catch-22.

As has already been noted, 30 states and the District of Columbia have approved the use of cannabis in medicine. California was the first in 1996, but THC was made available a decade earlier as a prescription drug with the trade name Marinol (dronabinol). Dronabinol was initially approved for treatment of the nausea and vomiting attendant on cancer chemotherapy. Its use was later expanded as an appetite stimulant in persons with AIDS or suffering from terminal cancer. A related cannabinoid, nabilone, has been on and off the market since the 1980s and is currently sold under the trade name Cesamet for nausea and vomiting.

Thirty years after the approval of dronabinol to ameliorate chemotherapy-induced nausea and vomiting, one might expect its place in medicine to be secure. It is not. The evidence available in 2015 in support of dronabinol for this purpose was judged to be of "low quality." I mention this because it is typical of virtually all proposed uses of cannabis in medicine.

Each comes with fervent supporters as well as skeptical critics from the medical establishment. As I noted earlier, the slow pace of arriving at definitive conclusions has much to do with the classification of marijuana as a Schedule I drug; many hope that this soon will be corrected with rescheduling.

Another source of confusion is that each state which has approved medical marijuana has its own list of conditions eligible for treatment. For example, in New York State, we have cancer, HIV/AIDS, Parkinson's disease, multiple sclerosis, spasticity from spinal injury, epilepsy, inflammatory bowel disease, Huntington's disease, and a variety of neuropathies. New York State does not permit the smoking of marijuana for medical purposes. In contrast, the California Compassionate Use Act 1996 explicitly identifies a number of conditions but concludes with "or any other illness for which marijuana provides relief." California, unlike New York, permits the smoking of medical marijuana. Finally, despite what individual states may do, medical use of marijuana remains illegal under federal law. Confusing indeed.

HOW DO WE KNOW WHETHER A DRUG WORKS?

The complexity of the endocannabinoid systems of the human body, together with our current rudimentary understanding of these systems, permits unlimited speculation as to possible beneficial and adverse effects of drugs acting upon them.[32] To illustrate the difficulties, both pharmacological and social, of the use of marijuana as a therapeutic agent, we will consider two conditions: epilepsy and pain. But before doing that, let us consider for a moment how it is that we know that a drug works. The proper therapeutic term is *efficacy*, the ability to bring about a desired effect.

If a drug is immediately life-saving and completely cures 100% of the patients treated, the determination of efficacy is easy. For most drugs, it is not so simple. For example, the National Institutes of Health in the United States spent hundreds of millions of dollars over a period of decades in proving, to nearly everyone's satisfaction, that drugs to reduce cholesterol save lives. The gold standard for such proof is the double-blind, placebo-controlled clinical trial in which neither the treating physician nor the patient is aware of the treatment given, and some patients are treated with a placebo, a pharmacologically inert substance. The code is broken only upon completion of the trial. The number of patients in the trial must be large enough to permit statistically based conclusions to be drawn.

The late Sir Archibald Cochrane was a Scotsman, a physician, and an epidemiologist who stressed the importance of randomized clinical trials. His name lives on in the form of Cochrane reviews, analyses of all available evidence regarding the merits of a given medical intervention; using statistical procedures, data from multiple studies are combined in what is called meta-analysis.

MARIJUANA AND EPILEPSY

In their review of the use of cannabinoids in the treatment of epilepsy, which appeared in the *New England Journal of Medicine* in September 2015, Daniel Freeman and Orrin Devinsky of New York University's Langone School of Medicine tell us that epilepsy was treated with cannabis as early as 1800 B.C. in what is now modern-day Iraq and that the use of cannabis for this disease flourished in Victorian England.[33] However, cannabis for epilepsy was largely supplanted by barbiturates in the early 20th century and later by Dilantin (phenytoin). (We will see more of barbiturates in chapter 5.) The Marihuana Tax Act of 1937 and the continued illegality of cannabis products further inhibited the use of cannabinoids.

It would be expected that the sedative and generally mellowing effects of marijuana would make it useful in a nonspecific way for any number of medical conditions. However, with the recognition that anandamide and the endocannabinoid systems play roles in the level of excitation of the nervous system and the fact that uncontrolled excitation with accompanying convulsions defines the ancient disease of epilepsy, it is plausible that THC and other cannabinoids might have a very specific and very powerful effect upon the condition. Indeed, recent decades have provided numerous anecdotal reports of efficacy. But, as has been said, the plural of anecdote is not data.

In their review, Drs. Friedman and Devinsky put it this way: ". . . despite the power of anecdote and the approval of cannabis by many state legislatures, only double-blind, placebo-controlled, randomized clinical trials . . . can provide reliable information on safety and efficacy. The use of medical cannabis for the treatment of epilepsy may go the way of vitamin and nutritional supplements, for which the science never caught up with the hype and was drowned out by unverified claims, sensational testimonials, and clever marketing."[34] A year earlier, the Cochrane group had said the following about cannabis and epilepsy:

No reliable conclusions can be drawn at present regarding the efficacy of cannabinoids as a treatment for epilepsy owing to the lack of adequate data from randomized, controlled trials of *delta*[9]-THC, cannabidiol, or any other cannabinoid.[35]

The American Academy of Neurology concurred with the Cochrane assessment.

AND THEN CAME THE CHILDREN

In 2016, Billy Caldwell was 10 years old and living in Northern Ireland. Billy suffered from severe epilepsy for which there seemed no remedy. All previous drug treatments had failed. His mother, in the hope that cannabis might be helpful, took Billy to Los Angeles, where he was treated with cannabis oil, a complex mixture extracted from *Cannabis sativa*. It contains both THC and cannabidiol (CBD), but various oils differ in the ratio of the two chemicals. Recall that THC acts primarily on CB_1 receptors, while the primary sites of action of cannabidiol are the CB_2 receptors. Thus, we might expect the effects of cannabis oil to be as complex as the mixture itself.

For Billy, the results were remarkable; according to his mother, he was seizure-free for months. Upon their return home to Northern Ireland, Billy received a prescription for cannabis oil to be made by a Dublin-based pharmaceutical house. The beneficial effects continued. Whimsically it was suggested that the oil be called "Billy's Bud." Billy's mother said that the family was "crying happy tears.[36] Those soon turned to tears of sorrow.

When officials in the Home Office, the ministerial department of the United Kingdom responsible for drug policy, learned of Billy's prescription, they had it halted. In desperation, Billy and his mother traveled to Canada, where they were able to obtain the needed cannabis oil. However, upon their return home via London's Heathrow Airport on June 11, 2018, the cannabis product was seized.[37]

The confiscation of Billy's cannabis oil met with widespread condemnation both in the media and by some politicians. Most important, Sajid Javid, Britain's home secretary, was sympathetic. Just 8 days after the Heathrow incident, Javid ordered a review of cannabis policy. In doing so, he said, "Recent cases involving sick children made it clear to me that our position on cannabis related medicinal products was not satisfactory."[38] At the same time, Javid ordered the immediate issuance of a limited license allowing the use of cannabis oil by Billy and by a second boy, 6-year-old Alphie Dingley. In Alphie's case, his family had moved to the Netherlands so that he could be treated with cannabis oil, a treatment which Alphie's parents characterized as "nothing short of a miracle."[39] In March 2018, for financial reasons, the family was obliged to return to the United Kingdom, where their multiple petitions for use of cannabis oil were denied. On July 26, 2108, shortly after the government's review of cannabis was completed, it was announced that cannabis-derived medicines were to be available for use by specialist clinicians in the United Kingdom by November 1, 2018.[40]

In those states of the United States in which medical marijuana had been approved, it was possible in theory to treat epilepsy with cannabis products. In practice, this did not often take place. In the absence of acceptable data to prove efficacy, few physicians were inclined to follow that therapeutic pathway. But parents of epileptic children did not have the luxury of waiting for proof.

In 2013, Brenda Porter and Catherine Jacobsen of the Department of Neurology of Stanford University School of Medicine conducted a survey of parents who had turned to cannabidiol-enriched cannabis to treat their children.[41] Eighty-four percent reported a reduction in seizure frequency. Prior to this, the average number of traditional anti-epileptic drugs which had been tried and failed was 12.

In an editorial accompanying the Porter and Jacobson article, Joseph Sirven of the Mayo Clinic College of Medicine said the following:

> . . . this study, if anything, highlights the failure of the health-care system as a whole to grapple with better management of epilepsy as it deals with our most vulnerable citizens—our children. Amazingly, like any good parents who want to ameliorate suffering in their kids, they have taken matters into their own hands delivering an unproven treatment without solid information on the safety and viability of medical cannabis for epilepsy. It is providential and positive that they have been able to receive benefit but tragic that they had to conduct their own trial without help in order to accomplish this.[42]

A glimmer of hope for children suffering two rare forms of epilepsy came with the completion in 2017 and 2018 of clinical trials which examined the efficacy of cannabidiol. Both trials were double blind and placebo controlled, thus meeting accepted criteria for proof of efficacy. The first, led by Orrin Devinsky, whom we met earlier in this chapter, tested the effects of CBD in 120 children afflicted with Dravet syndrome.[43] In this form of epilepsy, seizures usually commence in the early months of life. As the disease progresses, intellectual disability is often seen, and death is not uncommon. Traditional anti-epileptic drugs are ineffectual. Dr. Devinsky and his colleagues observed that, in a 14-week period of treatment with CBD, monthly seizure frequency was decreased by 50%; 6 of the children were seizure-free. In contrast, seizures were unabated during 4 weeks of placebo treatment.

The second clinical trial, also conducted by the Devinsky group and involving 30 treatment centers, examined the addition of one of two doses of cannabidiol to conventional anti-epileptic medication in a condition called Lennox-Gastaut syndrome.[44] In this form of the disease, seizures usually begin in the second to sixth year of life, are severe, and are often accompanied by cognitive impairment. More specifically, the investigators looked at the incidence of drop seizures in which there is very brief loss of muscle tone often involving the muscles of the neck. For the CBD doses of 30 mg and 20 mg, the reductions in drop seizures were 42% and 37%, respectively. These compare with a 17% reduction following placebo treatment. The improvement following CBD treatment compared with the placebo was statistically significant, that is, not likely to be due to chance variation.

Some might argue that these two clinical trials accomplished nothing more than to confirm previous anecdotal reports. But anecdotal accounts of benefits of CBD for epileptic children, however moving, had not resulted in action by the Food and Drug Administration of the United States. In contrast, the clinical trials, well designed, double blind, and placebo controlled, had a meaningful impact. On June 25, 2018, the Food and Drug Administration approved an oral solution of cannabidiol under the trade name Epidiolex for use in children and adults suffering from either the Dravet or Lennox-Gastaut syndromes.[45]

It is obvious that there is much more yet to be learned about the efficacy of cannabinoids in the treatment of epilepsy. Might the combination of THC and CBD in the cannabis oil so helpful to Billy Caldwell and Alphie Dingley be more effective than CBD alone? And if that is the case, what is the ideal ratio of THC to CBD? Too much THC and children will have hallucinations akin to those described by Gautier and Hollister.[46][47] Too little and perhaps efficacy will be diminished.

In an editorial accompanying the 2017 Dravet syndrome study, Samuel Berkovic of the University of Melbourne pointed out that CBD is not without adverse effects.[48] Among them are diarrhea, vomiting, fatigue, and fever. In some cases, these effects were sufficiently severe that some children dropped out of the study. Furthermore, it is obvious that CBD is not a magic bullet for Dravet syndrome; not all children responded to the treatment. A possible explanation pointed out by Dr. Berkovic is that Dravet syndrome is well understood to involve a single gene defect and that there is no evidence to suggest that CBD directly interacts with the neuronal consequences of that defect. This caveat does not, of course, in any way diminish the benefit received by the majority of children. How much more quickly these benefits might have been recognized had there not been decades-long restrictions on marijuana clinical research is unknowable.

MARIJUANA AND PAIN

There is no doubt that, over the course of several millennia, the soothing properties of cannabis have often been employed to alleviate pain. There is likewise no doubt that the efficacy of cannabis in relieving pain is inferior to that of the opioids. However, with the ever-rising incidence of opioid-related deaths, the thought has been entertained that cannabinoids might partially displace opioids in the treatment of chronic pain and thus blunt the effects of the "opioid epidemic." The great virtue of any such displacement is that THC does not kill in overdose.

The most extensively studied commercial cannabis-derived product for the relief of pain is nabiximols under the trade name Sativex.[49] It is a whole-plant extract containing both THC and CBD. It is administered as an oral spray. In 2005, Sativex was approved for use in Canada for the treatment of neuropathic pain in multiple sclerosis and pain due to cancer. Subsequently, approval came in the European Union, New Zealand, and Israel but, as of 2018, the product remained under review in the United States.

The evidence that cannabinoids may have a place in the treatment of chronic pain has steadily increased.[50,51,52,53] Equally important are data suggesting that the use of cannabis for this purpose may indeed ameliorate certain aspects of the opioid crisis in the United States and elsewhere. For example, studies of Medicare Part-D and Medicaid enrollees have found that per capita prescription of opioids is lower in those states in which medical marijuana is legal as compared with those states in which it is not.[54,55] More important, states with medical cannabis laws were found during the period 1999–2010 to have significantly lower opioid overdose mortality rates.[56,57] It must be noted that a subsequent investigation which extended analysis through 2017 failed to replicate the earlier conclusion that the availability of medical marijuana lowered opiate overdose deaths.[58] Nonetheless, Michael Barnes, writing in the *British Medical Journal* in 2015, expressed the view that "Allowing doctors to prescribe cannabis might prevent tens of thousands of opioid deaths worldwide each year."[59]

THE BENEFIT-RISK RATIO FOR MARIJUANA

For every drug for every malady, one must consider the benefit-risk ratio. If a cannabinoid were found to provide benefit for a given condition, we would then need to consider possible adverse effects. This is a reasonably straightforward exercise for a therapeutic effect, but what are we to do with recreational marijuana? Here the benefit is less well defined; some would even suggest that benefit in the form of pleasure derived from the use of a drug is immoral and justifies no risk whatsoever. In either case, recreational or therapeutic, the possible adverse effects are the same.

Nora D. Volkow, MD, has been the director of the National Institute on Drug Abuse since 2003. In an article in the *New England Journal of Medicine* in 2014, she expressed her views on the adverse health effects of marijuana and on, in her words, "the popular notion that marijuana is a harmless pleasure."[60] Listed as immediate effects are (a) impaired short-term memory, (b) impaired motor coordination, (c) altered judgment, increasing the risk of sexual behaviors that facilitate the transmission of sexually transmitted disease, and (d) paranoia and psychosis. With longer term or heavy use, Dr. Volkow cites (a) addiction, (b) altered brain development, (c) poor educational outcome, (d) cognitive impairment with lowered IQ, (e) diminished life satisfaction and achievement, (f) chronic bronchitis, and (g) increased risk of psychosis disorders, including schizophrenia.

As the availability of products containing higher concentrations of THC becomes more common, the risk of psychosis deserves special mention. Subsequent to Dr. Volkow's warning in 2014, the results of two studies were published by a group from the Department of Psychosis Studies at King's College London. In the first, which appeared in 2016, data were gathered from 10 previous studies involving 67,816 individuals. It was concluded that high levels of cannabis use produce a nearly four-fold increase in the risk of schizophrenia and other psychotic disorders.[61] While admitting that they could not unequivocally establish a causal relationship, the authors urged increased educational efforts aimed at particularly vulnerable persons, such as those with a family history of schizophrenia.

A subsequent investigation by the King's College group, published in 2019, found a relationship between the frequency of use and the potency of the cannabis preparations to the risk of psychosis.[62] The subjects were 901 patients who presented to psychiatric services in Europe and Brazil with first-episode psychosis. These were compared with control subjects from the same populations. Daily use of cannabis was associated with a three-fold increase in the probability of psychosis and, for those using high-potency THC preparations, that is, greater than 10% THC, the risk was nearly five times greater than for nonusers. In Amsterdam, a city in which cannabis has been widely available for many years, the investigators suggested that first-episode psychosis would be reduced by 50% in the absence of cannabis use. The authors close with these words: "Therefore, it is of public health importance to acknowledge alongside the potential medicinal properties of some cannabis constituents the potential adverse effects that are associated with daily cannabis use especially of high-potency varieties."

When speaking of addiction, Dr. Volkow mentions an increased risk of the use of other illicit drugs; this is the gateway hypothesis, the idea that, for example, the use of marijuana might lead to opioid addiction. This hypothesis emerged in the 1930s and has remained as a pillar of the anti-marijuana message. A definitive refutation of the gateway hypothesis is not at hand. Nonetheless, it seems reasonable that those who are immersed in a drug culture are more likely to sample and perhaps become addicted to a variety of other drugs. Indeed, reliable data indicate that young people who smoke nicotine-containing cigarettes are 15 times as likely as nonsmokers to move on to the use of marijuana.

PHYSICAL DEPENDENCE AND ADDICTION: POTHEADS

Well into the 1970s, standard textbooks of pharmacology expressed the view that physical dependence and addiction do not occur with marijuana use. However, in 1976, it was reported that, when experienced marijuana users were given THC every 4 hours around the clock, a withdrawal syndrome occurred. The syndrome was characterized by irritability, restlessness, insomnia, and loss of appetite. This constellation of signs and symptoms fully meets our definition of physical dependence provided in chapter 1.

Might addiction to marijuana occur as well? To answer that question, we must remind ourselves of my preferred definition of addiction as a behavioral state of compulsive, uncontrollable drug craving and seeking which does harm to the individual. The answer to our question will not be found in well-controlled clinical studies; conduct of such studies is ethically impermissible. Instead, we must depend upon anecdotal accounts from persons sometimes called "potheads." The story that follows is one such account.

Neal Pollack is the editor in chief of *Book and Film Globe* and the author in 2018 of an article describing his addiction and current recovery.[63]

When I had my first cup of coffee in the morning, I pressed the little button on my vape pen, waited for the blue glow, took a huge inhale and then blew it into the mug so that I could suck in the THC and the caffeine at the same time. Then I took another hit, and another. In the afternoons, I'd smoke a bowl, or pop a gummy bear, or both. At night, I got high before eating dinner or watching the ball game. Maybe I'd stop getting stoned a little bit before bed, but what was the point. If I went to bed high, I could just wake up high. . . . I spent years telling myself that marijuana isn't addictive, and so I didn't have a problem. But clearly I did. . . . My son was born in 2002. . . . I got stoned the day my son came home from the hospital and stayed that way, with a few breaks, for a decade and a half. Of course I put him in danger because I couldn't stop getting high. I was a drug addict. . . . In March of 2017, my mother died. . . . I was high when I watched her die, I was high at her funeral, and I was high every day for the next eight months. To say I was "self-medicating" to deal with grief would be too kind. My addicted self took grief as a no-limits license to get stoned.

In November 2017, Pollack purchased a ticket for baseball's World Series; it turned out to be fraudulent. "So high that I couldn't remember where I had parked, I started screaming outside the stadium . . . security guards surrounded me. I looked into a car mirror and saw an old man, sobbing over a baseball game. That was the moment I accepted that I had a problem. Three weeks later, I quit."

Pollack suffered no dramatic withdrawal syndrome; "a couple of twitchy nights" is how he described it. He was pleased to see how much he could accomplish when "75% of my life doesn't revolve around obtaining or consuming weed." His conclusion: ". . . marijuana addiction exists, and it almost wrecked my life."

Based upon the experience of Pollack and others like him, I believe that some among us will exhibit addiction to marijuana and that this addiction will be accompanied by adverse personal and social effects. The extent to which the prevalence of marijuana addiction will be increased by legalization of the drug for recreational use remains to be seen.

Just as was the case for each of the proposed beneficial effects of cannabis, each of the postulated adverse effects of marijuana use given by Dr. Volkow is worthy of serious scientific investigation. Only when both benefit and risk are adequately understood can a rational decision be reached as to the merits of either medical or recreational use. Clearly the voters in those states which have approved recreational or medical marijuana have reached a decision as to benefit and risk. The judgment of medical science will take longer.

A CANNABINOID FOR OBESITY?

I will close this section with a happier yet still unsatisfactory example of cannabinoids applied to human health. We have seen how THC in the form of Marinol is useful as an appetite stimulant for those with terminal cancer or AIDS. Even casual smokers of marijuana are familiar with "the munchies," cannabis-induced stimulation of appetite. These observations suggest a role for the endocannabinoid system in controlling food intake. If THC stimulates appetite by acting on CB_1 receptors in the brain, might we suppress appetite by producing an opposite effect on those same receptors? The answer to that question came in a drug called rimonabant with the trade name Acomplia.[64] Pharmacologically speaking, rimonabant does not block CB_1 receptors in a fashion like that of naloxone blocking opioid receptors. Instead, it is what is called an *inverse agonist*. Rimonabant acts to produce an effect opposite to that of THC. The hope was that rimonabant would provide a potent weapon in controlling obesity.

Rimonabant was approved for the treatment of obesity in England in 2006. Within 2 years, its use had spread to more than 50 countries and results were quite promising for weight loss. But, again, we must consider the benefit-risk ratio. Alas, disturbing reports of depression and thoughts of suicide began to appear in users.[65] It was for this reason that rimonabant was removed from the European market in 2008, and the drug was never approved for use in the United States.

THE FUTURE

As has been pointed by many before me, it is difficult to make predictions. Nonetheless, I will offer a few. Barring a major health crisis, legalization at the state level for both medical and recreational marijuana will continue apace. For example, in October 2018, Canada began a country-wide legalization of recreational marijuana. In the United States, as state and local governments where recreational use is permitted become more dependent on taxes raised from the cannabis industries, pressure will increase to alter federal prohibitions and to move marijuana from Schedule I to Schedule II. The latter will foster increased research into the consequences of chronic use, especially among the young. Edible marijuana products will present a particular hazard for infants and toddlers, and products appealing to children will be banned. Illicit laboratories around the world and in the United States will continue to discover and market for street use ever more potent and hazardous cannabinoids. Legitimate research will lead to better drugs with which to target the endocannabinoid system with the hope being that the promise of medical marijuana will be realized. However, as expressed by Leo Hollister nearly a half century ago, "It is unlikely that pharmacological answers will provide answers to social questions about cannabis."[66]

NOTES

1. National Center for Biotechnology Information (2017) The health effects of cannabis and cannabinoids: The current state of evidence and recommendations for research. https://www.ncbi.nlm.nih.gov/books/NBK425763/

2. European Monitoring Centre for Drugs and Drug Addiction (2017) United Kingdom drug report. http://www.emcdda.europa.eu/system/files/publications/4529/TD0116925ENN.pdf

3. Nahas G (1973) *Marihuana—Deceptive Weed*. New York: Raven Press Books.

4. Annas GJ (2014) Medical marijuana, physicians, and the law. *NEJM* 371(11):983–985.

5. Federal Bureau of Investigation Uniform Crime Reporting Program (2017) 2016 crime in the United States. https://ucr.fbi.gov/crime-in-the-u.s/2016/crime-in-the-u.s.-2016/cius-2016/topic-pages/persons-arrested?

6. Newton-Holmes G (2017) Cannabis as medicine. *BMJ* 357:j2130.

7. Todd AR (1946) Hashish. *Experientia* 2:55–60.

8. Gaoni Y, Mechoulam R (1964) Isolation, structure, and partial synthesis of an active constituent of hashish. *J Am Chem Soc* 86:1646–1647.

9. Devane WA, Dysarz FA, Johnson MR, Melvin LS, Howlett AC (1988) Determination and characterization of a cannabinoid receptor in rat brain. *Mol Pharmacol* 34:605–613.

10. Devane WA, Hanus L, Breuer A, Pertwee RG, Stevenson LA, Griffin G, Gibson D, Mandelbaum A, Etinger A, Mechoulam R (1992) Isolation and structure of a brain constituent that binds to the cannabinoid receptor. *Science* 258:1946–1949.

11. Pertwee RG (2015) Endocannabinoids and their pharmacological actions. *Handb Exp Pharmacol* 231:1–37.

12. Munro S, Thomas K, Abu-Shaar M (1993) Molecular characterization of a peripheral receptor for cannabinoids. *Nature* 365:61–65.

13. Schultes RE, Hofmann, A (1980) *The Botany and Chemistry of Hallucinogens*, 2nd edition. Springfield, IL: Charles C. Thomas.

14. Rietz R (1998) Self-experimentation. *JAMA* 280(23):2043.

15. Ebin D (1961) *The Drug Experience. First Person Accounts of Addicts, Writers, Scientists and Others*. New York: Orion.

16. Melges FT, Tinklenberg JR, Hollister LE, Gillespie HK (1970) Temporal disintegration and depersonalization during marijuana intoxication. *Arch Gen Psychiatry* 23(3):204–210.

17. Barrett FS, Schlienz NJ, Lembeck N, Wagas M, Vandrey R (2018) "Hallucinations" following acute cannabis dosing: A case report and comparison to other hallucinogenic drugs. *Cannabis Cannabinoid Res* 3(1):85–93.

18. Moreau J (1845) *Hashish and Mental Illness*. Paris: Masson; 1973 English translation by G. J. Barnett, edited by H. Peters and G. G. Nahas. New York: Raven Press.

19. Cushny AR (1913) *A Textbook of Pharmacology and Therapeutics*. Philadelphia: Lea & Febiger.

20. Udell GG (1972) *Opium and Narcotic Laws*. Washington, D.C.: U.S. Government Printing Office.

21. Udell GG (1972) *Opium and Narcotic Laws*. Washington, D.C.: U.S. Government Printing Office.

22. Anslinger HJ, Thompkins WF (1953) *The Traffic in Narcotics*. New York: Funk and Wagnalls.

23. Udell GG (1972) *Opium and Narcotic Laws.* Washington, D.C.: U.S. Government Printing Office.
24. First Report of the National Commission on Marijuana and Drug Abuse (1972) *Marihuana: A Signal of Misunderstanding.* Washington, D.C.: U.S. Government Printing Office.
25. Major's Committee on Marihuana (1944) *The Marihuana Problem in the City of New York—Sociological, Medical, Psychological, and Pharmacological Studies.* Lancaster, PA: Cattell.
26. Office of the Chairman (1982) *An Analysis of Marijuana Policy.* Washington, D.C.: National Academies Press.
27. New York Times Editorial Board (2016) Outrageous sentences for marijuana. *New York Times,* April 14.
28. Sessions JB (2016) Senate Caucus on International Narcotics Control SD-226, April 5.
29. Marcin T (2017) Wat Jeff Sessions has said about marijuana. *Newsweek,* March 28.
30. Heller J (1955) *Catch-22.* New York: Dell.
31. Udell GG (1972) *Opium and Narcotic Laws.* Washington, D.C.: U.S. Government Printing Office.
32. Kaur R, Ambwani SR, Singh S (2016) Endocannabinoid system: A multi-faceted therapeutic target. *Curr Clin Pharmacol* 11(2):110–117.
33. Friedman D, Devinsky O (2015) Cannabinoids in the treatment of epilepsy. *NEJM* 373(11)1048–1058.
34. Friedman D, Devinsky O (2015) Cannabinoids in the treatment of epilepsy. *NEJM* 373(11)1048–1058.
35. Gloss D, Vickrey B (2014) Cannabinoids for epilepsy. *Cochrane Database Syst Rev* 3:CD00920.
36. Pasha-Robinson L (2017) Billy Caldwell: Medical cannabis oil named after 11-year-old boy with severe epilepsy. *The Independent,* July 8.
37. Gayle D (2018) Medicinal cannabis: how two heartbreaking cases helped change the law. *The Guardian,* July 26.
38. Torjesen I (2018) Medical cannabis will be available on prescription in UK from autumn. *BMJ* 362:k3290.
39. Baker N (2018) Cannabis cure: Who is Alfie Dingley? *The Sun,* June 18.
40. Torjesen I (2018) Medical cannabis will be available on prescription in UK from autumn. *BMJ* 362:k3290.
41. Porter BR, Jacobson C (2013) Report of a parent survey of cannabidiol-enriched cannabis use in pediatric-resistant epilepsy. *Epilepsy Behav* 29:574–577.
42. Sirven Joseph I. (2013) Medical marijuana for epilepsy: Winds of change. *Epilepsy Behav* 29:435–436.
43. Devinsky O, Cross JH, Laux L, Marsh E, Miller I, NabboutR, Scheffer IE, Theile EA, Wright S. (2017) Trial of cannabidiol for drug-resistant seizures in the Dravet Syndrome. *NEJM* 376 (21):2011.
44. Devinsky O, Patel AD, Cross H, Villaneuva V, Wirrell EC, Privitera M, Greenwood SM, Roberts C, Checketts D, VanLandingham KE, Zuberi SM (2018) Effect of cannabidiol on drop seizures in the Lennox-Gastaut Syndrome. *NEJM* 378:1888–1897.
45. Food and Drug Administration (2018) Press Release, June 25.
46. Ebin D (1961) *The Drug Experience. First Person Accounts of Addicts, Writers, Scientists and Others.* New York: Orion.

47. Melges FT, Tinklenberg JR, Hollister LE, Gillespie HK (1970) Temporal disintegration and depersonalization during marijuana intoxication. *Arch Gen Psychiatry* 23(3):204–210.

48. Berkovic SF (2017) Cannabinoids for epilepsy—real data, at last. *NEJM* 376(21):2075–2076.

49. LeafScience (2018) What is Sativex (nabiximols)? https://www.leafscience.com/2017/11/02/what-is-sativex-nabiximols/

50. Whiting PF, Wolff RF, Deshpande S et al. (2015) Cannabinoids for medical use: A systematic review and meta-analysis. *JAMA* 313:2456–2473.

51. Hill KP (2015) Medical marijuana for treatment of chronic pain and other medical and psychiatric problems. *JAMA* 313(24):2474–2483.

52. Davis MP (2016) Cannabinoids for symptom management and cancer therapy: The evidence. *J Natl Compr Canc Netw* 14(7):915–922.

53. National Academy of Sciences, Engineering, and Medicine. (2017) *The Health Effects of Cannabis and Cannabinoids*. Washington, D.C.: National Academies Press.

54. Wen H, Hockenberry JM (2018) Association of medical and adult-use marijuana laws with opioid prescribing for Medicaid enrollees. *JAMA Intern Med* 178(5):673–679.

55. Bradford AC, Bradford WD, Abraham A, Adams GB (2018) Association between US state medical cannabis laws and opioid prescribing in the Medicare Part D population. *JAMA Intern Med* 178(5):667–673.

56. Bachhuber MA, Saloner B, Cunningham CO, Barry CL (2014) Medical cannabis laws and opioid analgesic overdose mortality in the United States. 1999–2010. *JAMA Intern Med* 174:1668–1673.

57. Powell D, Pacula RL, Jacobseon M (2018) Do medical marijuana laws reduce addictions and deaths related to painkillers? *J Health Econ* 58:290–42.

58. Shover CL, Davis CS, Gordon SC, Humphreys K (2019) Association between medical cannabis laws and opioid overdose mortality has reversed over time. *Proc Natl Acad Sci USA*. https://doi.org/10.1073/pnas. 1903434116, Epub ahead of print.

59. Barnes MP (2018) The case for medical marijuana. *BMJ* 2018;362:k3230 doi: 10.1136/bmj.k3230

60. Volkow ND, Baler RD, Compton WM, Weiss SRB (2014) Adverse health effects of marijuana use. *NEJM* 370(23):2219–2227.

61. Marconi A, Di Forti M, Lewis CM, Murray RM, Vassos E (2016) Meta-analysis of the association between the level of cannabis use and risk of psychosis. *Schizophrenia Bulletin* 42(5):1262–1269.

62. DiForti M, Quattrone D, Freeman TP, et al. (2019) The contribution of cannabis use to variation in the incidence of psychotic disorder across Europe (EU-GEI): A multi-center case-control study. *The Lancet Psychiatry*, March 19 (epub ahead of print).

63. Pollack N (2018) I'm just a middle-aged dad addicted to pot. *New York Times*, October 6.

64. Van Gaal LF, Rissanen AM, Scheen AJ, Ziegler O, Rössner, S (2005) Effects of the cannabinoid-1 receptor blocker rimonabant on weight reduction and cardiovascular risk factors in overweight patients: 1-year experience from the RIO-Europe study. *The Lancet* 365:1389–1397.

65. Christensen R, Kristensen PK, Bartels EM, Bliddal H, Astrup A (2007) Efficacy and safety of the weight-loss drug rimonabant: a meta-analysis of randomized trials. *The Lancet* 370:1706–1713.

66. Hollister LE (1969) Criminal laws and the control of drugs of abuse. An historical view of the law (or, it's the lawyer's fault). *J Clin Pharmacol* 9(6):345–348.

CHAPTER 4

ᴄⱱᴏ

Stimulants

From Coca to Caffeine

Unlike the opiates, which are a rather homogeneous group, the drugs we call stimulants come in a variety of forms. In this chapter, we will devote most of our time to the classical stimulants, cocaine and the amphetamines, but will consider as well caffeine, nicotine, ephedrine, and modafinil. All are capable of enhancing mental and physical performance, and some produce distinctly pleasurable effects that sometimes lead to addiction.

About the time that humans living in what is now South America started to draw on the walls of their caves, one among them discovered the unusual properties of the coca shrub.[1] When the leaves were chewed, wondrous things happened to the chewer: Hunger and fatigue were replaced by feelings of strength and power; the world seemed not such a bad place to live. By the time Francisco Pizarro led his conquistadors into Peru early in the 16th century, coca leaf had found an exalted place in the Incan Empire. One legend has it that coca was brought from heaven to earth by Manco Capac, son of the Sun god and the Inca from whom the ruling class traced its lineage. (Interesting how often royalty has claimed divine origins.)

The Spaniards developed no great respect for coca, regarding it as but another facet of a pagan people who had no claim on civilization. But the new rulers were nothing if not practical. Coca allowed native workers to be pushed beyond the normal bounds of physical endurance. More tin and silver could be brought from the mines with fewer workers fed less food.

Our Love Affair with Drugs: The History, the Science, the Politics. Jerrold Winter, Oxford University Press (2020). © Jerrold Winter.
DOI: 10.1093/oso/9780190051464.001.0001

Coca leaf lost its status as a sacrament and a pleasure of the ruling class. It became a part of the internal economy of Spanish Peru, a means of enhancing productivity, and a contributor to the destruction of the Incan people and their civilization.

It was inevitable that Europeans would become familiar with the effects of coca leaf both by their observation of native use and by personal experience. In 1859, an Italian physician named Paolo Mantegazza who had spent some time among the Peruvian natives put it this way.

> Some of the images I tried to describe in the first part of my delirium were full of poetry. I sneered at the poor mortals condemned to live in this valley of tears while I, carried on the winds of two leaves of coca, went flying through the spaces of many worlds, each more splendid than the one before. An hour later I was sufficiently calm to write these words in a steady hand: God is unjust because He made man incapable of sustaining the effect of coca all lifelong.[2]

Mantegazza was not the first or the last to describe the effects of coca in glowing terms. Why then in the nearly four centuries from Pizarro to Mantegazza did its use not spread throughout Europe? Some have suggested that deterioration of coca leaf in its long trip from the New World to the Old left a generally inactive material. What was needed was a wedding of the ancient coca leaf with modern chemistry.

THE COCA LEAF YIELDS COCAINE

A year before Dr. Mantegazza wrote in praise of coca leaf, Albert Niemann was accepted as a student in the laboratory of Friedrich Wohler, one of Germany's most distinguished chemists. The master assigned to Niemann the task of isolating pure chemicals from coca leaf. Just 2 years later, Niemann submitted his PhD dissertation to the faculty. It was entitled "Uber eine neue organische Base in den Cocablattern" (Concerning a New Organic Base in Coca Leaf).[3] Niemann gave the name *cocaine* to the substance he had purified. Coca's modern era had begun.

Freed of the constraints and uncertainties imposed by crude coca leaf, scientists in many parts of the world began to explore the pharmacological properties of cocaine. Reports of its value in treating tuberculosis, stomach problems, impotence, and various mental disturbances became common. American physicians recommended cocaine as a cure for alcoholism and for the "opium habit." If these claims seem extravagant, keep in mind that medicine of the mid-19th century was still largely the practice of the placebo effect. A drug with the properties described by Mantegazza would be expected to have ascribed to it great healing powers.

One who sought to capitalize on the powers of cocaine was Angelo Mariani, a Corsican chemist.[4] In 1862, he offered for sale *Vin Tonique Mariani*. Mariani's wine was a Bordeaux containing coca leaves. The alcohol did a good job of freeing the cocaine from the leaves. An advertisement of the day made the expected claims that the wine would improve the health of the user. Meanwhile, in the United States, similar tonics appeared. One was Pemberton's French Wine, which gave birth in 1885 to a nonalcoholic derivative with the name Coca-Cola. Today's Coca-Cola is flavored with coca leaves from which the cocaine has been removed and caffeine added to provide a stimulant effect.

FREUD MEETS COCAINE

The reports of cocaine's medical uses were read by a young Viennese physician named Sigmund Freud who was then just starting his career. He was eager to make his mark, and the study of cocaine seemed a likely means. In addition, several of the proposed uses of cocaine were of direct personal interest; Freud often suffered both indigestion and depression. Using himself as a subject, he began his observations on cocaine. In June 1884, he published an article, "Uber Coca," which he described to his fiancé as "a song of praise to this magical substance." Freud's enthusiasm was unbounded.

> I take very small doses of it regularly against depression . . . with the most brilliant success. The effects are exhilarating and lasting euphoria, which in no way differs from the normal euphoria of a healthy person. . . .You perceive an increase in self-control and possess more vitality and capacity for work.[5]

In addition, Freud advocated the use of cocaine in digestive disorders, as an appetite stimulant, in morphine withdrawal, for asthma, and as an aphrodisiac.

Two of Freud's colleagues at the Vienna General Hospital soon provided evidence for the blessings as well as the sorrows of cocaine use. Albert Niemann had noted in his thesis of 1860 that cocaine, when tasted, produced a numbness of the tongue. This observation was largely ignored, though some, including Freud, commented on the possible use of cocaine as a local anesthetic. However, more than two decades would pass before Carl Koller gained lasting fame when he reported to the German Ophthalmological Society in 1884 that cocaine applied to the eye causes complete anesthesia.[6] He had observed this phenomenon first in animals, then in himself, and finally in patients on whom he performed surgery. That was a blessing conferred by cocaine. The use of the drug for the treatment of morphine addiction did not work out quite so well.

A second of Freud's Viennese colleagues, Ernst von Fleischl-Marxow, was a distinguished medical scientist and much admired by Freud. However, in 1871, after conducting an autopsy, von Fleischl-Marxow had developed an infection that ended in the amputation of his thumb. Nerves at the site of the amputation became inflamed and caused constant pain. In seeking relief, von Fleischl-Marxow was soon physically dependent on morphine.[7] In an attempt to help his friend, Freud told him of the reports from America of the use of cocaine in morphine dependence. (It turned out that these reports were largely the work of two American companies, Merck and Parke-Davis, who marketed a variety of cocaine products.)

At first, things went well. Von Fleischl-Marxow was slowly weaned from morphine; he was no longer physically dependent upon it. Freud thought that he had made a great discovery. The honeymoon soon ended. It became apparent that von Fleischl-Marxow was as addicted to cocaine as surely as he had been to morphine.

From what we have so far been told by Mantegazza and by Freud, chronic use of cocaine should be far preferable to that of morphine. It is not. Von Fleischl-Marxow soon was injecting large amounts of the drug. While cocaine maintained its power to produce euphoria, crushing depression quickly followed, alleviated only by more cocaine. Freud's earlier statement that there is "absolutely no craving for the further use of cocaine" became, for von Fleischl-Marxow, a mockery. But cocaine held other surprises for Freud and his patient.

Von Fleischl-Marxow began to appear insane. We now call the condition "cocaine psychosis."[8] The departure from reality which chronic use of cocaine causes has some peculiar features. The user becomes paranoid. Suspicious and fearful of people and things, there is a tendency to take violent action against them. Tactile hallucinations are common. Of von Fleischl-Marxow, Carl Koller said, "many a night have I spent with him watching him dig imaginary insects out of his skin." At the time of his death at age 45 and just 7 years after his first experience with cocaine, von Fleischl-Marxow was still dependent upon "this magical substance."

Freud soon gave up his advocacy of cocaine. His experience with von Fleischl-Marxow coupled with condemnation of his stand by others in the scientific community was enough to cause him to move on to the nonpharmacological areas of medicine for which he is best remembered.

But others remained faithful; the use of cocaine both in medical and in nonmedical settings increased in Europe and in this country for the next 20 years or so.

THE COCAINE HABIT

On the cusp of the 20th century, patent medicines containing cocaine were freely available in any drugstore. One European example was called "Forced March." Marketed by Burroughs Welcome & Company, it contained both cocaine and caffeine. Intended to promote mental and physical endurance, the product accompanied both Robert Falcon Scott and Ernest Shackleton in their expeditions to the South Pole.[9]

However, by the early 1900s a number of factors combined against free access to cocaine. Evidence accumulated regarding the hazards of addiction, cocaine psychosis, and the possibility of death. The American Medical Association was becoming more powerful and more insistent that not everyone who wished to do so should practice medicine and prescribe drugs. And there were elements of racism and of hysteria; apocryphal accounts of white women raped and killed by black men crazed by cocaine or marijuana found a receptive audience. The Harrison Narcotics Act of 1914 removed cocaine from patent medicines; henceforth, only with a physician's prescription could cocaine be obtained. Eight years later, cocaine was legally defined, together with morphine and heroin, as a narcotic.[10] This triumph of political action over pharmacological fact introduced still another element of confusion regarding the true properties of cocaine.

Meanwhile, in the United States, a vigorous discussion of, as one author put it, "the so-called cocaine habit," was taking place among physicians. Writing in the *New York Medical Journal* in 1886, William Alexander Hammond, a leading neurologist, described his cocaine experiences "with exuberance" and likened it to the "coffee habit."[11] Others were not so sanguine, noting hallucinations and delusions and, upon discontinuation, depression and despondency. Some were convinced of the reality of cocaine addiction. In our discussion of addiction in chapter 1, I suggested that its roots are multiple and often intertwined. A New York physician, writing in 1887, said " . . . take a man who is ill, down-hearted, unable to work, and subject him to the cocaine experience, and what would become of him? Would he not be in imminent danger of becoming a cocaine addict?"[12] A reminder that, to be original, you must not read; it has all been said before.

WILLIAM HALSTEAD'S COCAINE ADDICTION

The report by Carl Koller of the use of cocaine as a local anesthetic in eye surgery caught the attention of William Stewart Halsted, a leading New York City surgeon, who began to explore the use of cocaine for regional anesthesia. To do this, he injected cocaine into himself and his students and traced the areas of local anesthesia which resulted. They soon extended their observations to include dental surgery and a variety of minor surgical procedures. However, in the words of Dr. Gerald Imber, Halsted's biographer, " . . . the medical students and their teachers came to enjoy the sense of exhilaration they experienced in the experiments, and began to use cocaine snuff and injections in social circumstances." None less than Halsted himself who soon developed cocaine addiction. His condition was manifest by disorganized writing and a deterioration of his professional activities. Encouraged by his colleagues, he eventually entered a private hospital where, over the course of 7 months, his treatment included morphine in a mirror image of Freud's substitution of cocaine for the morphine addiction of von Fleischl-Marxow. For the remainder of his illustrious life, which included brilliant surgical innovations and the founding with three others of the Johns Hopkins University School of Medicine, Halsted maintained a morphine addiction punctuated with bouts of cocaine use.[13]

COCAINE TOLERANCE, PHYSICAL DEPENDENCE, AND ADDICTION

What then can be said about cocaine with respect to tolerance, physical dependence, and addiction? Tolerance is variable, studies in animals even provide evidence that some effects may be enhanced with continued use, and there is no classical withdrawal syndrome as seen with depressant drugs such as the barbiturates, alcohol, and the opiates. However, most now recognize a cocaine withdrawal syndrome characterized by depressed mood, impaired concentration, fatigue, and insomnia. With respect to addiction, Dr. Sidney Cohen, chief of psychosomatic medicine at the Veterans Administration Hospital in Los Angeles, wrote in 1975 that "tolerance and withdrawal do not occur, therefore it is incorrect to speak of cocaine addiction."[14] This statement depends of course on a definition of addiction that includes a dramatic withdrawal syndrome. However, addiction defined as I have suggested to you, a behavioral state of uncontrolled, compulsive drug craving and seeking with harm to the individual, is surely met by the experiences of Drs. Halsted and von Fleischl-Marxow. But let us consider a contemporary example of cocaine addiction.

". . . a healthy 20-year-old man with a 4-year history of cocaine addiction," identified only as "Mr. R," was described by Dr. Eileen E. Reynolds, to an audience at Beth Israel Deaconess Medical Center in Boston.[15] Mr. R's own words may be difficult to comprehend for those who have not experienced the power of addictive drugs, but they will ring true for any who have:

> I don't remember the first time I smoked crack cocaine. It puts you [in] another world. I can't explain the euphoric feeling that it gives you, but it's a feeling I had never experienced before. I just want to sit there and enjoy the feeling and not think about anything or do anything. I have to keep doing it constantly to keep up the high. . . . I was smoking about five times a week and lost my apartment. . . . Everything was falling apart with my relationship, and I was beginning to miss work a lot. But I just couldn't control it. You know, it overtook me. That's all I thought about and all I wanted to do was to keep smoking. Everything else was secondary . . . I had been in a treatment program for five months, then a half-way house; I got a job. . . . And one night, I wanted to smoke. I just said, "I want to smoke again. I want that feeling again." . . . Hopefully when my life is, you know, if it ever comes to that point where I have a family and I have the career I want, I won't need that escape or need that extra feeling. I'll be high on life, you know, just . . . naturally.

CRACK COCAINE

Mr. R refers to smoking "crack cocaine." Here we must consider a little more pharmacology. A substantial part of the controversy about the goodness or the badness of cocaine, whether in the 19th or the 21st century, results from a failure to appreciate the ways in which cocaine's effects are altered by the form of cocaine used and the route which cocaine takes to get from outside my body to my brain. Generally speaking, the intensity of cocaine's effects, the "height of the high" among other things, is determined by these factors. And there is good reason to believe that the higher my cocaine high, the greater the probability that I will lose control of my use of cocaine; that I will become a cocaine addict.

Recall Albert Niemann's PhD dissertation: "Concerning a New *Organic Base* (my emphasis) in Coca Leaf." A weak organic base is a chemical that changes its form depending upon the acidity of its environment. When acid is present, cocaine forms a salt; when acid is absent, cocaine occurs as a "free base." The form of cocaine that is used, free base or salt, is one factor in the effects that are produced.

Until fairly recently, cocaine as used in this country was cocaine hydrochloride, a salt. In its pure form, it is a beautiful white crystalline substance. Cocaine salt snorted into the nose is slowly changed to the free base that is then absorbed across the nasal membranes, enters the blood, and is carried to the brain; it is a relatively slow process but fast enough to produce an acceptable high. A hazard of this route of administration is that cocaine constricts the blood vessels of the nose with eventual tissue destruction that may progress to perforation of the nasal septum.

In the Olympics of drug use, it is the height of the high that counts. A means to increase the height is to increase the rate at which cocaine reaches the brain. One way is to inject cocaine salt under the skin ("skin popping") or directly into a vein ("main-lining"). A second is to use cocaine in its basic form rather than as a salt. To obtain the free base, one simply dissolves cocaine hydrochloride in water and adds a layer of ether and an alkali such as sodium hydroxide. The salt is changed to the free base, which then moves from the water to the ether. Evaporate the ether and you have free base cocaine. This conversion of salt to base is not without its hazards; ether is very volatile and very flammable; more than one free baser has learned that by experience.

Cocaine base is a pasty substance rather than a lovely crystal but with certain virtues of its own. Primary among these is that, unlike the salt, which decomposes if heated, free base cocaine can be smoked. While we usually think of our lungs only as a way to get oxygen into our blood and carbon dioxide out, the enormous surface area of the lungs also provides a very efficient means to absorb drugs like cocaine (and nicotine and the THC of marijuana). The height of the high following the inhalation of vaporized free base cocaine rivals that of intravenous injection.

One final note on the forms of cocaine. In 1986, the press began to tell us about "crack" or "rock," variously described as a new kind of cocaine or a new derivative of cocaine, one with much greater power to induce dependence than the old cocaine. That same year, a federal sentencing guideline was passed mandating 5 years in prison for possession of 5 grams of crack cocaine by a first-time offender. The same sentence for possession of cocaine hydrochloride would require 500 grams. In 1989, a young black woman in Texas was sentenced to life imprisonment without the possibility of parole for conspiracy to distribute crack cocaine. These disparities in the penalties associated with crack cocaine and cocaine hydrochloride have no basis in science; they are the same drug.

In fact, crack is free base cocaine obtained without bothering with the ether step. A water solution of cocaine hydrochloride is made alkaline and the free base, being water insoluble, sinks to the bottom and is collected. The emergence of acquired immune deficiency syndrome (AIDS) and its association with the injection of illicit drugs has made the smoking of cocaine base much more attractive to serious cocaine users. In addition, many who would not consider the intravenous use of drugs willingly smoke crack. Thus exposed to the highest of cocaine highs, a significant number will lose control of their use and are properly called addicts.

THE SYMPATHETIC NERVOUS SYSTEM

The discovery of the pharmacological properties of the coca leaf and the isolation of cocaine by Albert Niemann were remarkable human achievements. But it was Mother Nature, through countless millennia of evolution, who provided the physiological system upon which cocaine acts. When one of our ancestors was confronted by a lion or an alligator or perhaps a nasty human carrying a club, that branch of the nervous system called the sympathetic was activated. The main messengers of the sympathetic nervous system are adrenaline (epinephrine), noradrenaline (norepinephrine), and dopamine. Acting at multiple sites, these chemicals increase heart rate and the volume of blood pumped; more air flows through the lungs and more blood is directed to our muscles. Just as we would be today, the sympathetic nervous system made our ancestor ready either to flee or to fight. Drugs like cocaine, which replicate these effects, are called sympathomimetics. Other prominent members of the sympathomimetic family, which we soon will discuss, are the amphetamines.

As we already have seen for cocaine, sympathomimetic drugs also act directly upon the brain. If sleepy, we become alert. If fatigued, we become energized. A significant mediator of these effects is an increase in levels of dopamine. Brain circuits in which dopamine serves as the neurotransmitter are intimately involved in all manner of pleasure: food, drugs, sex, rock and roll, you name it, all trigger release of dopamine. In chemically mimicking these naturally occurring pleasurable events, sympathomimetics such as cocaine and the amphetamines can induce euphoria, a major contributor to their addictive properties.

We have all heard stories of persons, often elderly, who have dropped dead of a heart attack or stroke upon being confronted by an intruder or upon greeting a long lost relative. Is there such a thing as dying of fright or happiness? Indeed, there is. The human heart depends on a wonderfully orchestrated series of electrical and mechanical events to maintain its rate and rhythm. In times of intense fear or joy, the sympathetic nervous system increases the rate and force of contraction of the heart; the blood pressure rises as the arteries constrict. A normal heart responds to excitement or exercise or stimulants in a reliable and predictable fashion. There is a smooth acceleration of rate and force. Raised blood pressure sends more blood to where it's needed. A diseased heart and weakened blood vessels are another matter. A vessel may burst or the heart may fall into dysrhythmic and unproductive activity. Just as exercise or excitement sometimes ends in sudden death, so too may the use of cocaine or an amphetamine.

For those with heart disease, stimulants are much more hazardous than for the rest of us. Unfortunately, we must sometimes define "a diseased heart" after the fact. The death of a basketball player named Len Bias in June of 1986 is an example.[16] Len Bias was by all the usual criteria a healthy young man, just 22 years of age and destined to have a professional basketball career. Yet the facts seem to be that he snorted cocaine (or, some say, smoked crack cocaine) and was soon dead. After the fact, we can say that his heart was unusually susceptible to the disorganizing effects of cocaine—little comfort to Len Bias or his family. Stimulant-induced sudden death due to stroke or heart attack is a rare event but one which should give pause even to casual users of these drugs

THE AMPHETAMINES

Earlier I mentioned the naturally occurring chemicals in our brains that act upon receptors for opiates and upon receptors for THC. These are the endorphins and the endocannabinoids, respectively. In a similar fashion, playing a role in the sympathetic nervous system, is phenethylamine (PEA). You have not heard of PEA as a drug, although we might expect it to be cocaine-like in its actions. That it is not is probably due to its very short duration of action. However, a very simple modification of PEA yields amphetamine, a chemical possessed of a long duration of action and perfectly suited to both medical and recreational use. All that we have learned about cocaine is applicable to amphetamine and to its close chemical cousin, methamphetamine. Testifying to the power of methamphetamine are the words of the writer and recovering addict Nic Sheff following his first encounter with the drug: "There was a feeling like—my God, this is what I've been missing my entire life. It completed me. I felt whole for the first time." Sheff spent the next 4 years, in his words, " . . . chasing that first high. I wanted desperately to feel that wholeness again."[17]

BENZADRINE, DEXADRINE, AND STEREOCHEMISTRY

Though first synthesized in 1887, amphetamine did not find a medical use until several decades later when the American pharmaceutical firm Smith, Kline & French patented the Benzedrine inhaler for the treatment of asthma and nasal congestion. The inhaler contained dl-amphetamine, oil of lavender, and menthol. Not long after its introduction, recreational pharmacologists noted that one could easily extract the amphetamine from the inhaler for use as a cocaine substitute. For Smith, Kline & French, such diversion into illicit use represented but a tiny market. Broader medical applications were needed.

In the late 1920s, Gordon Alles, a California chemist and pharmacologist, had investigated the ability of amphetamine to ease the breathing of asthmatics and, in 1932, had patented two amphetamine salts for that purpose. But Alles recognized something else: the cocaine-like mood-elevating properties of the amphetamines. He approached Smith, Kline & French with his ideas and, in 1937, dl-amphetamine in pill form was marketed as Benzedrine Sulfate. Soon thereafter came Dexedrine Sulfate (d-amphetamine) and Desoxyn (d-methamphetamine hydrochloride).

Now I want to digress briefly, say a little more about organic chemistry, and tell you of one of the peculiarities of the amphetamines. It derives from the nature of the chemical bonds formed by carbon. Human life on this planet is carbon based. Each carbon atom is able to connect with four other elements in forming the ever more complex structures of our bodies and of all other animals and plants. These chemical bonds have direction in space.

Imagine a pyramid with four faces, a tetrahedron, and imagine a carbon atom in its center with bonds pointing out to each of the four points of the pyramid. Label the base points A, B, and C, with D being the top of the pyramid. If we were to swap the positions of the bonds to yield A, C, B at the base, we would now have two nonsuperimposable structures; they are mirror images just as are your left and right hands. Likewise, d-amphetamine and l-amphetamine are mirror images; they are called isomers of one another.

But the drug receptors we talked about in chapter 1 have three-dimensional structures as well, and it is a general principle of pharmacology that drug and receptor must establish intimate contact if an effect is to be produced. Thus, as far as the receptor is concerned, d-amphetamine and l-amphetamine are two different drugs. Think of trying to put your left hand into your right glove or your right foot into your left shoe. It just wouldn't be a very good fit. This is the reason why, in speaking of the amphetamines and other drugs, we may see the prefix *d-* for dextro (right) and *l-*for levo (left). An example of when both isomers are present is *d,l*-amphetamine. The configuration in space of a drug may have quite dramatic consequences. For example, *d*-methamphetamine is a very effective stimulant which often leads to addiction. In contrast, *l*-methamphetamine is so benign that is can be used in nasal decongestants such as the Vick's Vapor Inhaler and sold without a prescription. (The seller, Procter and Gamble, lists the ingredient as *levmetamfetamine*.)

AMPHETAMINES ARE BROUGHT TO THE MASSES

Advertisements for the amphetamines, first directed at America's physicians and later at the general public, were extravagant; the American housewife was a frequent target.[18] Physicians were advised that "many of your patients, particularly housewives, are crushed under a load of dull, routine duties that leave them in a state of mental and emotional fatigue— Dexedrine will give them a feeling of energy and well-being, renewing their interest in life and living." Recalling that cocaine of the coca leaves allowed the natives of Peru to get along with less food, the similar appetite-suppressant effects of amphetamines were employed to treat obesity. In one advertisement, a Rubenesque woman says, "Oh, dear, this diet is getting me down." The answer proffered "for the patient who is all flesh and no willpower" was d-amphetamine. It "does more than curb appetite but will reawaken mental alertness and optimism." For the menopausal woman, Dexedrine would "restore the savor and zest for life" so that "Now she can cook breakfast again."[19] Men were not ignored. Accompanying a picture of a tweed-clothed man, cigarette in hand, consulting his golf pro, is the comment that "For the patient who resigns himself to mere existence during the middle period of life, depression can easily get the upper hand. The seemingly endless, daily routine of living is approached with apathy, inertia, and lack of interest . . . for such a patient, Dexedrine Sulfate is of unequalled value."

The ability of sympathomimetic drugs to counter fatigue and increase endurance, effects which had been noted by Sigmund Freud, did not go unnoticed by the military.[20] During Germany's Blitzkrieg of 1939–1940 in which Poland, the Netherlands, Belgium, and France were overrun, it is estimated that 35 million tablets of methamphetamine, known to the Germans as Pervitin, were issued to ground troops and pilots. After conducting a series of laboratory and field tests with amphetamine purchased from Smith, Kline & French, Britain's Royal Air Force began in 1942 to issue the drug to crews of Bomber Command. Bernard Montgomery, famed for his defeat of Erwin Rommel in tank battles at El Alamein, was a particular advocate of amphetamine use and issued it to all in his Middle East group. Following experiments in medical students at Northwestern University, the US military made amphetamine available to all theater commanders in early 1943. General Dwight Eisenhower, then Supreme Commander of the North African Theater of Operations, requested 3 million tablets. By the end of the war, Smith, Kline & French alone was producing 365 million amphetamine pills a year with other providers, bringing the total to twice that number. Stimulant use by the US military has continued to this day, in war and in peace.

Gordon Alles and Smith, Kline & French had created the first drug for what Peter Kramer would many years later call *cosmetic psychopharmacology*, the idea that a drug can make you feel better than normal yet still normal. For two decades, the amphetamines were legal, inexpensive, and available without a prescription. Adverse effects, including scattered deaths, were largely ignored; amphetamine psychosis, closely resembling the cocaine psychosis of von Fleischl-Marxow, was identified as early as 1938. Nonetheless, amphetamine became for many the modern way to get high. The eclipse of cocaine was nearly complete. The use of cocaine soon was confined largely to the decadent rich and a few jazz musicians.

In 1959, with signs of an amphetamine epidemic on the horizon, the Food and Drug Administration banned Benzedrine inhalers and ruled that a physician's prescription for amphetamines was required. The Comprehensive Drug Abuse Prevention and Control Act of 1970 placed amphetamines in Schedule II, along with cocaine and morphine, with added regulation of the 50 tons of amphetamine produced that year. Federal and state laws were enacted; in Georgia, mere possession of methamphetamine called for imprisonment for 2 to 15 years with a second offense upping the penalty to as much as 30 years. Ironically, these moves to control the amphetamines appear to have played a major role in the rebirth of cocaine use in the decades of the 1970s and 1980s.

ATTENTION-DEFICIT HYPERACTIVITY DISORDER

Sales of Benzedrine in the 1930s for the treatment of asthma and other respiratory disorders, Parkinson's disease, depression, narcolepsy, and obesity were impressive, but Smith, Kline & French remained eager to establish still other markets. One possibility was as a means to enhance academic performance in children. Smith, Kline & French provided free samples of

Benzedrine to any physician who wished to test the idea. However, the results of a few small trials were unimpressive, and Smith, Kline & French soon abandoned the efforts.

Charles Bradley had other ideas. He was the medical director of the Emma Pendleton Bradley Home in Providence, Rhode Island. The home had been created in 1931 by a bequest from his great-uncle and great-aunt and named for their daughter. Stricken with encephalitis at the age of 7, Emma Bradley suffered from epilepsy, learning difficulties, and cerebral palsy. The Bradley Home was the nation's first neuropsychiatric hospital for children. Still in operation today, the Home, in accordance with George Bradley's will, gives free care to poor children of Rhode Island.

Dr. Bradley's primary interest was in the behavioral disorders of children of normal intelligence. Pneumoencephalography, which involves the draining of cerebrospinal fluid, was a routine part of his medical work-up. Unfortunately, the children often suffered severe headaches following the procedure. Bradley reasoned that an increase in the production of cerebrospinal fluid might prevent the headaches and that the stimulant effects of Benzedrine might accomplish that end.

Bradley was mistaken; Benzedrine did not diminish the headaches. However, in publishing his results in 1937, he wrote the following:

> The most striking change in behavior occurred in the school activities of many of these patients. There appeared a definite drive to accomplish as much as possible. Fifteen of the thirty children responded to Benzedrine by becoming distinctly subdued in their emotional responses. Clinically in all cases, there was an improvement from the social standpoint.[21]

Over the course of the next dozen years, Bradley continued his studies, adding Dexedrine as a treatment option. Summarizing his work in 1950, he reiterated his belief that in children of normal intelligence with symptoms of "restlessness, noisiness, hyperactivity, and distractibility," stimulant drugs could produce "striking improvement in school adjustment and academic performance."[22] His work and his conclusions were largely ignored by the medical community. How then have we reached the point where, in 2016, some 6 million American children aged 4–17 years received a diagnosis of attention-deficit/hyperactivity disorder (ADHD) and nearly 4 million of these children were prescribed a stimulant drug?[23] Part of the answer to our question lies in the evolution of the term "ADHD." Its origins are in a series of lectures delivered in 1902 by Sir George Still to the Royal College of Physicians in London.[24] He described children who had difficulty with self-control and attention to tasks at hand, often resistant to discipline. He attributed this behavior to a defect in "moral control" by which he meant an inability to conform to social standards. More specifically, he identified "a quite abnormal incapacity for sustained attention." In the years that followed, others attributed such behavior to head trauma, encephalitis, or mental retardation. These studies were most often conducted in psychiatric hospitals, as were those of Bradley. The American Psychiatric Association in 1952 attached the label "minimal brain dysfunction" to the syndrome. Over the years the label evolved first into "hyperkinetic reaction of childhood," then into "attention deficit disorder with or without hyperactivity," until finally in 1964 and reaffirmed in 2013, the term "attention-deficit/hyperactivity disorder" was agreed upon.

ADHD was to be a psychiatric disorder, and psychiatric labels are seldom popular. Cancer will buy you sympathy; mental illness, not so much. But at least "ADHD" was a more palatable term than "minimal brain dysfunction." Nonetheless, the notion that ADHD should, as Bradley had suggested in 1937, be treated with amphetamines, met with vigorous condemnation. Exposure of children to drugs associated with addiction, death, psychosis, and social transgressions was simply unacceptable to physicians and parents. Something else accounts for the current enthusiasm both for the diagnosis of ADHD and for the use of stimulant drugs in its treatment. That something else, I would suggest to you, is the magic of marketing.

Only two countries in the world, New Zealand and the Unites States, permit the direct advertising of prescription drugs to the general public. Thus, beginning in 1997, American parents were exposed to advertisements on television and in the print media telling them of ADHD and its treatment.[25] Appeal often was made to the insecurities of parenthood; one ad led off with "I am not a bad Mom" and continued with "Now there is a new way to help him out." Another said, "The mean child doesn't mean it" and went on to ask, "Is he a hyperactive problem child?" Accompanying a picture of a young boy in a monster costume was the suggestion that he could be converted "from a monster to a loveable child." Emphasis was placed on school work: "Reveal his potential," "Improves academic performance," "Schoolwork that matches his intelligence," "Today I got a good mark." Advertisements such as these were nearly always directed at the parents of male children, reflecting the fact that boys are two to three times more likely than girls to receive a diagnosis of ADHD and are up to nine times more likely to be referred for evaluation and treatment, often with a stimulant.

THE RISE OF RITALIN AND ADDERALL

Amphetamines retained their unsavory reputation, so pharmacological alternatives were needed. New drugs are attractive to us by virtue of offering superior benefits with diminished adverse effects. For ADHD, the new drugs were given the trades names Ritalin and Adderall. The chemical name for Ritalin is methylphenidate. An extended-release form is now sold as Metadate and Concerta. First synthesized in the laboratories of Ciba, a Swiss pharmaceutical house, during World War II, methylphenidate was introduced to the scientific community in 1954 as "a central stimulant with a new chemical constitution." Over the next two decades, reports appeared supporting its use to treat depression, narcolepsy, Parkinson's disease, behavioral problems of old age, anxiety, and fatigue, to improve athletic performance, and to suppress appetite. In children, numerous studies suggested amphetamine-like efficacy in treating the spectrum of symptoms we now call ADHD.

If my description of the uses of methylphenidate sounds familiar, it is because we have already seen amphetamines used for all of these indications. But Ritalin was said to be different. In a Ciba advertisement it was described as "a new, mild, smooth-acting antidepressant and stimulant chemically *unrelated to the amphetamines*" (my emphasis). In treating ADHD, being "unrelated to the amphetamines" had appeal for physicians aware of the dangers of amphetamines and for parents unwilling to have their children treated with these much-feared drugs.

It is true that the chemical structure of Ritalin is more complex than that of amphetamine. However, embedded within that structure is methamphetamine. Thus, we should not be surprised that Ritalin possesses all of the properties of methamphetamine. Indeed, in addition to its suggested medical uses, adverse effects, including psychosis and addiction, closely resemble those of cocaine, amphetamine, and methamphetamine. Nonetheless, the implication that Ritalin is distinctly different from the amphetamines in treating ADHD proved useful for marketing. Our second "new" drug for the treatment of ADHD is Adderall. Here I need not tell you of the pharmacological effects of Adderall but only to list its ingredients. Adderall combines *d*-amphetamine, *l*-amphetamine, and *d,l*-amphetamine. Adderall is simply an irrational mixture of amphetamines. Earlier we saw *d,l*-amphetamine as Benzedrine and *d*-amphetamine as Dexedrine.

The serendipitous discovery by Charles Bradley some 80 years ago that many children suffering what we now call ADHD has led to the widespread use of amphetamine and amphetamine-like drugs in these children. However, controversy continues to surround both the diagnosis of ADHD and the use of stimulants. There are regular calls in the medical community for reexamination of both treatment and diagnosis. Methylphenidate and the amphetamines, we are reminded, have all of the properties of cocaine. In explaining the remarkable increase in the incidence and treatment of ADHD, I mentioned increased awareness of the condition coupled with extensive marketing efforts. But there is another factor: stimulants work. When part of a comprehensive plan of treatment, these drugs bring benefit to many children with a valid diagnosis of ADHD.

The emphasis placed by many advertisements on the ability of stimulants to improve schoolwork did not go unnoticed. Recall that Smith, Kline & French had suggested this possibility back in the 1930s. Today, many parents actively seek the ADHD label, and stimulants, for their teenagers in the hope that test scores, including those on the SAT, will improve. Some physicians have gone so far as to prescribe stimulants to poor children without a valid diagnosis of ADHD in the hope that the multiple effects of poverty on learning will be overcome.[26] This practice is an entirely legal example of what is called "off-label prescribing." Any Food and Drug Administration–approved drug can be prescribed for any condition by any licensed physician but cannot be advertised for other than approved purposes. The extent that this is done with stimulants is unknown and may be unknowable in that few physicians are likely to admit to the practice.

One concern about the use of stimulants in children with ADHD is that they may be more susceptible to stimulant abuse in later years. These fears have not been borne out in follow-up studies. But what of the non-ADHD child or adolescent given these drugs in an attempt to improve academic performance? I am unaware of data that address this issue, but the story told by Cat Marnell in her 2017 memoir *How to Murder Your Life* gives us pause.[27]

Growing up in an affluent suburb of Washington, D.C., Cat's father, a psychiatrist, prescribed Adderall to help her with her school work. A side effect much appreciated by the teenager was suppression of her appetite. In the years that followed, Cat continued her use of Adderall. At age 26, she was a 5 foot, 4 inch, 97 pound, associate beauty editor at *Lucky*, a fashion magazine aimed at young women. In describing her addiction, she wrote, "I was always strung out on Adderall . . . How much Adderall was I always strung out on, you ask? Lots of Adderall. Enough Adderall . . . to suppress all the appetites of all the starving children in all the world!"

ATTENTION-DEFICIT/HYPERACTIVITY DISORDER:
NOT JUST FOR CHILDREN ANYMORE

ADHD was long thought to be a childhood condition that disappeared with the onset of puberty. However, beginning in the 1970s, reports began to appear suggesting that this might not be the case. Indeed, the current consensus is that ADHD persists into adulthood for perhaps 60% of those diagnosed as children. Adding to the number of those who suffer what is now called adult ADHD are those in whom the signs were not identified or treated in childhood. Overall, it is estimated that 4% of the adult population suffers from the condition.[28]

What defines adult ADHD? Might you or I have it? The Mayo Clinic tells us that "the main features of ADHD may include difficulty paying attention, impulsiveness and restlessness . . . everyday tasks can be a challenge. Adults with ADHD may find it difficult to focus and prioritize, leading to missed deadlines and forgotten meetings or social plans. The inability to control impulses can range from impatience waiting in line or driving in traffic to mood swings and outbursts of anger."[29] With that spectrum of symptoms, it is not surprising that diagnoses for adult ADHD increased 35% in the period 2009–2013. Sales of stimulant drugs, already brisk, increased still further. By 2017, adult ADHD accounted for nearly one half of all stimulant prescriptions. The increases for women were particularly dramatic with a five-fold increase in stimulant prescriptions over the period 2003 to 2015.[30]

A cynic might suggest that, in the age of the Internet, self-diagnosis of adult ADHD followed by consultation with a physician provides a convenient and legal way to obtain an amphetamine or methylphenidate prescription for the mood-enhancing, work-promoting, fatigue-combating effects of the drugs. Many of us are aware of individuals who have done precisely that.

AMPHETAMINES AND THE ATHLETE

From what I've already told you about the effects of cocaine and the amphetamines, it may have occurred to you that athletic performance might be improved by these drugs. And indeed it is. That fact was established nearly six decades ago in a group of collegiate swimmers by Henry K. Beecher, professor of anesthesiology at Harvard Medical School. Following modest doses of amphetamine, the swimmers improved their times by 1% to 2%.[31] Not a lot, you might say, but the difference between winning and losing in competition can be very slight indeed. For example, in the 2016 Rio Olympics, swimmer Mark Horton of Australia won the men's 400 meter freestyle event by 0.13 seconds over Su Yang of China. That's a difference of just 0.06%. Given the promise of even a slight gain in performance and given the very significant financial rewards to be had, it is not difficult to understand why many athletes have been tempted to use stimulants.

An interesting outbreak of adult ADHD occurred in major league baseball in 2007. Amphetamines have been a part of major league baseball for several decades; 2 years after his retirement in 2001, Hall of Fame outfielder Tony Gwynn estimated that 50% of players of his era used them, often in the form of Adderall or Ritalin.[32] At the time the league banned amphetamines for general use in 2006, 35 players had "therapeutic use exemptions," which permitted treatment of adult ADHD. The following season that number jumped to 111, fully 8.2% of the active players, two to four times the incidence in the general population.[33] We might wonder if exceptional talent in baseball is a risk factor for adult ADHD or if something else is working here.

MA HUANG TO METH LABS

We have seen something of the ancient history of opium, marijuana, and coca and the isolation of morphine, tetrahydrocannabinol, and cocaine, respectively, from them. I want now to tell you of another plant and the chemical it yields. Ephedra, known to many by its Chinese name *Ma Huang*, is an herb which has been used in Chinese medicine as a stimulant, as an anti-asthmatic, and to reduce fever for more than 5,000 years.[34] During colonial times in America, ephedra tea was recommended for colds, kidney disorders, and venereal diseases.

The Meiji era in Japan began in 1868 and with it came the opportunity for Japanese citizens, often with the support of the government, to visit the West. One of these was a 27-year-old physician named Nagayoshi Nagai. His destination was Germany, where he intended to seek further medical training, but he soon fell under the spell of August von Hofmann, professor of chemistry at the University of Berlin. Trained in traditional Chinese medicine, Nagai was quite familiar with Ma Huang. Just 4 years after his arrival, Nagai isolated from the herb the drugs ephedrine and its isomer pseudoephedrine. He noted that their pharmacological properties resembled those of adrenaline, one of our brain's chemicals that stimulate the sympathetic nervous system, and suggested that the drugs, because of their longer duration of action, might be useful in treating asthma.[35] Beginning in the 1920s, large amounts of ephedrine were produced in China and in Germany for export to the United States, and dozens of products containing ephedrine soon were marketed to the general public. Recognizing its medical value, a council of the American Medical Association in 1926 approved the use of ephedrine for the treatment of asthma, hay fever, bronchitis, emphysema, pertussis, shock, nasal congestion, and as an antidote for narcotic drugs—all of the uses we would expect for a sympathomimetic stimulant. In addition, the amphetamine-like ability of ephedrine to suppress hunger, elevate mood, and increase energy did not go unnoticed. The drug soon gained favor with those wishing to lose weight, with bodybuilders, and with exercisers of all kinds. For the latter purposes, ephedrine-containing products such as Bronkaid and Primatene are still today widely promoted on the Internet.

Recognizing the abuse liability of ephedrine, the Food and Drug Administration in the early 1990s considered regulation of the drug, but largely due to legal challenges and lobbying efforts on the part of marketers, no new rules were issued. Nonetheless, many commercial products were modified by replacing ephedrine with its less stimulant isomer pseudoephedrine. Familiar names among these were Allegra D, Benadryl Plus, Claritin-D, and the aptly named Sudafed.

Ephedrine remains a medically useful drug. For example, in spinal anesthesia, the inadvertent numbing of certain nerves may cause the patient's heart rate and blood pressure to fall to unacceptable levels. Ephedrine provides the anesthesiologist with an effective remedy. Nonetheless, ephedrine and pseudoephedrine would have remained little more than useful but largely unrecognized components of myriad over-the-counter cough, cold, and flu remedies were it not for the rise of methamphetamine as a drug of abuse.

Guided by recipes readily available on the Internet, thousands of amateur chemists, many in the hills and valleys of rural America, converted both ephedrine and pseudoephedrine into d-methamphetamine. Addictive use of methamphetamine has no geographical confines, but communities in Indiana, Kentucky, Tennessee, and Missouri were hit particularly hard. The federal response took the form of the Combat Methamphetamine Epidemic Act of 2005.[36] The Act did not ban the sale of products containing ephedrine or pseudoephedrine but established rules for record keeping, identification of buyers, and limits on daily and monthly amount that can be purchased. Between 2006 and 2010, seizures of clandestine laboratories declined significantly. Unfortunately, Mexican drug cartels soon took up the slack. By 2017, methamphetamine deaths were 18-fold greater than they had been at the turn of the century; in San Francisco in 2017, methamphetamine took more than twice as many lives as did heroin.[37]

NICOTINE

Two of the three stimulants with which we will close this chapter are well known to all. I refer to caffeine and nicotine. The third, modafinil, is more obscure but promises to offer an alternative to the amphetamines with fewer adverse effects.

Nicotine is a rather strange drug to find in this chapter. It differs in many respects from the stimulants we have discussed so far. Many people, on first smoking a cigarette, are nauseated by it. Extract the nicotine from a half dozen cigars and you have enough of the drug to cause death, yet there is little evidence that nicotine per se, in modest doses, causes ill health. Contrast this with the fact that nicotine in its association with the smoking of tobacco results in more deaths than all other drugs, licit and illicit, combined.

The *British Medical Journal* for December 13, 1952, included an article by Richard Doll and A. Bradford Hill entitled "A Study of the Etiology of Carcinoma of the Lung."[38] Based on interviews with 1,488 patients with lung cancer and an equal number of persons without the disease, they concluded that "the association between smoking and carcinoma of the lung is real." Unfortunately, nearly 30 years would pass before the Surgeon General of the United States was fully onboard: "Cigarette smoking is the single most important preventable environmental factor contributing to illness, disability, and death in the United States." Today it is estimated that 90% of all lung cancer results from the smoking of tobacco products. To this we may add cancer of the kidney and bladder as well as chronic obstructive pulmonary disease. And one need not be a smoker to be affected. Tony Gwynn, mentioned earlier regarding the use of amphetamines, died in 2014 at the age of 58 from cancer of the mouth and salivary glands. He attributed his disease to his long-time use of chewing tobacco.

It is true that a great deal has been accomplished in educating the public regarding the hazards of tobacco. In 1965, 42% of Americans smoked. By 2017, the prevalence had fallen to 14%. But the decrease has not been uniform across the population; smoking continues to afflict the most vulnerable. For those living in poverty, the rate is twice that of the more affluent. It is even worse for the homeless, 75% of whom smoke. Education matters as well: College graduates are four times less likely to smoke than those whose education ended with a GED.[39] My sentiments regarding tobacco were nicely expressed by an anonymous author in *The Lancet* who wrote that "Renewed effort . . . is needed to put tobacco where it belongs: in the history books, as a sad and strange episode in the story of human health."[40]

In our story of cocaine, we had to leave unnamed the Incan who discovered the intoxicating nature of coca. Likewise anonymous is the first person to experience the psychoactive properties of the tobacco plant. The natives of what are now Mexico and South America were chewing and smoking tobacco when the European explorers first arrived. We do know the names of the two men who introduced the plant and its uses to Europe.

In 1559, Jean Nicot was France's ambassador to Portugal. Upon his return to Paris, he brought to the court of the newly crowned King Francis II the seeds of a flowering garden plant which would later be given the name *Nicotiana* by the great Swedish taxonomist Carl Linnaeus. Nicot believed that the leaves of the plant, tobacco, had medicinal properties perhaps even as a shield against the plague. Beyond medical uses, tobacco soon came to be used as a recreational drug by members of the court and the upper levels of French society. It was King Francis who introduced the habit of snuff-taking. Others preferred to smoke tobacco, usually in a pipe. Through the efforts of Walter Raleigh, the court of Elizabeth I of England was soon to follow. But, with the death of Elizabeth and the coronation of James I, Sir Walter's fortunes declined. James disapproved of both tobacco and Raleigh, the latter disapproval ending with the loss of Raleigh's head in the Tower of London. With the support of the Royal College of Physicians, James launched the first antismoking campaign in the early 17th century.

With the isolation of nicotine from tobacco in 1828, it became possible to begin to unravel its pharmacological properties. In parallel with the sympathetic nervous system of which we spoke earlier, we have a cholinergic nervous system with acetylcholine as its transmitter. In addition, acetylcholine serves as the chemical link between nerve and muscle. Normally the synthesis, storage, release, and degradation of acetylcholine is nicely controlled. However, a lethal dose of nicotine, by overstimulating cholinergic receptors, causes paralysis of muscle and cessation of breathing. Though their mechanisms of action differ, nicotine shares this property with VX, the nerve gas believed to have been used in 2017 in the killing of the half-brother of Kim Jong-un, the president of North Korea. VX blocks the degradation of acetylcholine and, like nicotine, overstimulates the cholinergic receptors. Ironically, drugs similar to VX with the trade names Cognex and Aricept are used to treat memory loss in Alzheimer's disease. There is a modest degree of support for the use of nicotine in treating ADHD and for the memory and attention deficits of Alzheimer's disease.

The ability of nicotine to improve human cognitive performance has been well established using a variety of tests, often involving vigilance and fatigue. The drug is effective in nonsmokers as well as in smokers, but in the latter group we have the added benefit of allaying the nicotine withdrawal syndrome. Prominent in the syndrome are irritability, anxiety, difficulty concentrating, and depressed mood. In a fascinating study, the only one of its kind, combat pilots of the Hellenic Air Force who were pack-a-day smokers were evaluated after a 12-hour abstinence from smoking.[41] Tests administered immediately after completion of a flight revealed decrements in visual vigilance and mental arithmetic calculations as well as self-reported symptoms of withdrawal. The authors' conclusion was that, while pilots should be encouraged to stop smoking, in the meantime, avoidance of the withdrawal syndrome is highly desirable. Let us for a moment consider that syndrome as described by a man attempting to stop smoking.

> Daniel Davies met with his uncle for lunch. He had not seen him for a while and now Daniel thought that he looked tense, fidgety, haggard, jittery. His uncle quickly explained: "It's the worst withdrawal I've ever suffered" and he went on to say that he couldn't sleep, couldn't concentrate, couldn't think about anything else. "It is affecting my work, my marriage, his daily piece of mind."[42]

I have said that physical dependence is not addiction but, once physical dependence is established to nicotine, avoidance of the withdrawal syndrome is a powerful incentive to continue smoking. As I noted in chapter 1, once you have been tormented by the withdrawal syndrome, mere relief becomes delight. As a graduate student, I listened to a lecture by Douglas Riggs, MD, who was then chairman of the department in which I studied. Dr. Riggs was an ex-smoker and passionately opposed to the practice. After telling us of the pharmacology of nicotine, he closed his lecture with these words: "Don't sell your tobacco stock; you are betting on an addiction." Despite decades of denial by the tobacco industry, smokers are addicts as surely as are heroin users. Indeed, as I noted earlier, on a statistical basis, a heroin addict has a better chance of getting off his drug than does a smoker.

Given the undeniable adverse consequences of cigarette smoking, why has it been so difficult to erase smoking from our society? An obvious factor is of course the physical dependence that develops to nicotine. But there is more than that. Youthful rebellion is one element and the glamour of Hollywood films, past and present, continues to work its wonders. No lover of classic movies can forget Jerry Durrance in *Now, Voyager* as he puts two cigarettes to his lips, lights both, and hands one to Charlotte Vale. Perhaps we should be reminded that lung cancer took the lives of many of the stars of those films; Gary Cooper, Paul Newman, Yule Brenner, and John Wayne readily come to mind.

In a book simply called *Nicotine*, Gregor Hens, a German author, says that

> Every cigarette that I've ever smoked served a purpose—they were a signal, medication, a stimulant or a sedative, they were plaything, an accessory, a fetish object, something to help pass the time, a memory aid, a communication tool or an object of meditation. Sometimes . . . all at once.[43]

If some among us are destined to become nicotine addicts, how are we to treat the condition? Perhaps the answer lies in allowing the addiction to continue but delivering the nicotine by means less harmful than smoking.

In the early 1970s, shortly after methadone maintenance was introduced, it occurred to Murray Jarvik, a physician-scientist at UCLA, that a similar substitution might be useful for smokers. At the time, his wife, Lissy, who was, like her husband, a distinguished physician-scientist, was struggling to overcome her nicotine addiction. Aware of the ease with which nicotine penetrates the skin, Murray Jarvik and a colleague patented what came to be known as "the patch," a device to provide a low, constant dose of nicotine to the addict, thus avoiding the abstinence syndrome as well as the hazards brought on by the inhalation of tobacco smoke.[44] Introduced as a prescription medication in 1992, the nicotine patch became available over the counter in 1996. A companion product, nicotine chewing gum, permits absorption of nicotine across the mucous membranes of the mouth.

An alternative to the delivery of nicotine via patches applied to the skin are devices that vaporize nicotine and deliver the drug directly to the lungs as in the smoking of a cigarette. The advantage to the nicotine addict is that the carcinogenic combustion products of tobacco are avoided. While there is considerable hope that so-called e-cigarettes will have major health benefits for smokers, it seems likely as well that many nonsmokers will become physically dependent on nicotine and, in effect, addicted to vaporized nicotine. The recent development of devices capable of efficiently delivering nicotine in this fashion, Juul being the best known of the group, has led to an explosive increase in so-called vaping among adolescents. Virtually unknown in 2011, by 2018 more than a quarter of high school students in the United States were vaping.[45] The public health consequences of a dramatic increase in nicotine addiction, especially among the young, remain to be established.

CAFFEINE

The fact that caffeine is found in a variety of plants on several continents is remarkable. What is still more remarkable to me is that so many people, so long ago, in so many parts of the world discovered the virtues of these plants as a source of stimulation. From Africa comes the kola nut, used since prehistoric times in religious ceremonies. In what is now Central America, South America, and Mexico, the cocoa bean, yerba mate, and guarana were in use long before European colonization; indeed, the history of cocoa and chocolate extends back several thousand years. Relative newcomers are tea of 7th-century China and coffee in 15th-century Yemen. Since then, of course, the use of tea and coffee has spread around the world with the former as the national drink of England and coffee represented by Starbucks on 12,000 or so street corners of America.

Although various caffeine-containing brews have been in use for medicinal purposes for a thousand years or more, it was only with the isolation of caffeine from coffee in 1821, that the drug could takes its place in Western medicine. In medical texts of 19th-century America, caffeine was recommended as an antidote in opium and alcohol poisoning and to stimulate urine flow in what was then called dropsy, the collection of fluids, edema, as occurs in congestive heart failure. Over the years, better drugs were developed and one hardly finds mention of caffeine in a modern textbook of medicine. One use which has remained is to stimulate breathing. Thus, caffeine remains the drug of choice for this purpose in infants born prematurely.[46]

The psychoactive effects of caffeine were not ignored. More than a century ago, it was written by Arthur Cushny, professor of pharmacology in the University of London, that caffeine induces "a brightening of the intellectual faculties and an increased capacity for mental and physical work . . . ideas become clearer, thoughts flow more easily and rapidly, and fatigue and drowsiness disappear . . . a distinct benefit in intellectual work."[47]

Richard Ben Cramer won the Pulitzer Prize for international reporting in 1979. His obituary in The New York Times in 2013 was written by Margalit Fox.[48] In it, she says that "he ritually began his day with five cups of coffee, purchased en masse from the (Baltimore Sun) cafeteria, lined up on his desk and drunk in quick caffeinated succession." Caffeine is the most widely consumed stimulant drug in the world, and I feel safe in saying that nearly every reader of these words has consumed caffeine today in the form of tea, coffee, chocolate, or a soft drink. Making consumption of caffeine even more likely is the rise of "sports," "performance," and "energy" drinks. Most of these are witches' brews of sugar, B vitamins, and various exotic ingredients. But make no mistake, Red Bull, Rockstar Energy, Monster Energy, 5-Hour Energy, and virtually all the rest depend on caffeine for any significant effects. No-Doz and Vivarin are just plain caffeine and much cheaper.

More than a century ago, March 16, 1912, to be exact, a brief item in the *Journal of the American Medical Association* summarized studies of caffeine on "mental and motor efficiency."[49] One of the tasks employed was typewriting; both speed and accuracy were improved. Similar beneficial effects were observed in other mental and physical tasks and, with the exception of a slight decrement in holding the outstretched hand steady, no adverse effects were noted.

What have we learned about caffeine in the last 100 years? Well, we now talk with confidence about its mechanism of action. In chapter 1, I introduced you to the concept of the drug receptor. Caffeine acts primarily on the adenosine receptors of the brain.[50] These systems exert a generally suppressive effect on nervous activity and are thought to play a major role in sleep. The ability of caffeine to counter fatigue and prolong wakefulness is thus due to a blockade of elements of the adenosine system. In addition, there is convincing evidence that caffeine, again acting via adenosine, enhances the release of dopamine, one of the neurotransmitters via which cocaine and the amphetamines act.[51]

Having mentioned the amphetamines in the same sentence with caffeine, it is important that we compare and contrast them. With respect to performance-enhancing and anti-fatigue effects, the World War II studies that I mentioned earlier often found them to be quite comparable in improving the ability of a fatigued subject to maintain attention to a task. For these purposes, caffeine is a remarkably effective drug.

In chapter 1, I described the related phenomena of drug tolerance, physical dependence, and addiction. Do those who regularly ingest caffeine become tolerant to the effects of the drug? Yes, to a moderate degree. No harm is done. Does physical dependence accompany this tolerance? Yes. The classic withdrawal symptom for caffeine is headache often accompanied by irritability. Is it appropriate to speak of coffee drinkers as caffeine addicts?[52] As always, the answer depends on our definition of addiction. By the criteria of the definition I provided in chapter 1, the answer is "no" for the vast majority because no physical harm is done despite the presence of physical dependence. However, the latest edition of *The Diagnostic and Statistical Manual of Mental Disorders* of the American Psychiatric Association has a section called "Caffeine-Related Disorders" in which a withdrawal syndrome is recognized.[53] What really sets caffeine apart as a stimulant is the response of our society to it. Unlike cocaine and the amphetamines, we do not put people in jail for the use or sale of caffeine. But, as we have seen before, it is the dose that makes the poison.

Beginning in 2006, there began to appear scattered accounts of fatalities in Canada and the United States related to caffeine ingestion in the form of energy drinks. By the end of 2012, the Food and Drug Administration had received reports of about two dozen deaths associated with the use of drinks such as 5-Hour Energy, Red Bull, and Rockstar Energy Drink. The number of emergency room visits involving energy drinks doubled between 2007 and 2011. In about half of these, alcohol or another drug was taken in combination with the energy drink.[54]

The complex interaction between drugs and underlying disease states is illustrated by the death in 2011 of Anais Fournier, a 14-year-old Maryland girl.[55] She consumed about 48 ounces of Monster Energy Drink over a 2-day period. The medical examiner attributed her death to the toxic effects of caffeine on her heart. That much Monster Energy Drink contains about 500 mg of caffeine, roughly the amount in Richard Ben Cramer's five cups of coffee. However, unlike Mr. Cramer, Anais suffered from a genetic disorder in which connective tissue is defective. Science cannot decide the respective roles in her death of that disease state, the caffeine, or their combination. The lesson for all of us is that the heart, especially an aged or diseased heart, is not an organ to be trifled with.

A recent basis for optimism regarding coffee drinking comes from a huge study conducted under the auspices of the National Institutes of Health and the American Association of Retired Persons (AARP).[56] After excluding persons with pre-existing cancer or heart disease or who had previously suffered a stroke, the investigators ended up with 402,260 men and women aged 50 to 71. A questionnaire was completed and the participants were then followed for 14 years. During that period, there were 52,515 deaths (13%).

First the bad news: Coffee drinkers, both men and women, were more likely to die. However, coffee drinkers were also more likely to smoke cigarettes, less likely to exercise, and ate fewer fruits and vegetables. Now the good news: When the role of smoking, exercise, and diet were excluded by statistical methods, coffee drinkers had a reduced risk of death due to heart or lung disease, stroke, diabetes, and infection; incidence of cancer was unchanged. About one third of the subjects drank decaffeinated coffee and were equally well protected, thus suggesting that the essential factor in coffee may be other than caffeine. In concluding their 2012 report in the *New England Journal of Medicine*, Neal Freedman and his colleagues said this: "Our results provide reassurance with respect to the concern that coffee drinking might adversely affect health."

MODANIFIL

Narcolepsy is a condition in which a person may have a sudden onset of sleep sometimes accompanied by hallucinations. As was noted earlier, amphetamines have been used extensively in the treatment of narcolepsy but, as with all other applications of these drugs, there is concern about adverse effects, including addiction.

Michel Jouvet, who, until his death in 2017, was emeritus professor of experimental medicine at Claude Bernard University in Lyon, France, devoted his professional life to the study of sleep and its disorders and published a number of popular books on the subject. It was thus not surprising that an alternative stimulant, modafinil, would be brought to his attention by its French discoverers. In the mid-1980s, Professor Jouvet reported that modafinil was effective in narcolepsy.[57] The US Food and Drug Administration approved the drug for that condition in 1998 to be sold by Cephalon, an American pharmaceutical house, with the name Provigil. Later the Food and Drug Administration allowed its prescription for night shift workers and for excessive sleepiness associated with obstructive sleep apnea. In 2009, with the patent protection running out on Provigil, Cephalon introduced a closely related drug, armadafanil, under the trade name Nuvigil. A third member of the family is adrafanil, sold online with the name Olmifon.

Modafinil remains a bit of an enigma in terms of its mechanism of action. Initially it was thought to act in a fashion distinct from that of cocaine and the amphetamines. However, more recent studies suggest that it, like the amphetamines and cocaine, increases levels of dopamine and norepinephrine, the neurotransmitters intimately involved with pleasure, addiction, and alertness. In 2009, Nora Volkow, director of the National Institute on Drug Abuse, and her colleagues at Brookhaven National Laboratory, provided evidence in human subjects that modafinil acts in a fashion much more like cocaine and the amphetamines than had been suspected. She went on to call for "heightened awareness for potential abuse and dependence . . . in vulnerable populations."[58]

Although the use of modafinil is now widespread, there are few reports of adverse effects and little to suggest that it is cocaine-like in its abuse liability. The Drug Enforcement Administration has placed it in Schedule IV, meaning that it has accepted medical uses and a low potential for abuse. Many in the military believe that it provides a reasonable alternative to the amphetamines in sustaining alertness. Suggestions for the use of modafinil range from attention-deficit disorder, in both children and adults, to schizophrenia, treatment of stimulant abuse, and as an antidote for age-related memory impairment. Efficacy in none of these conditions has been proven. Nonetheless, I look forward to careful studies of each of these proposed uses.

MORE QUESTIONS THAN ANSWERS

Cocaine, amphetamine, methamphetamine, methylphenidate, caffeine, nicotine, and modafinil: We have covered a lot of ground with a chemically and mechanistically diverse group of drugs. They are united, however, in that each can, under appropriate circumstances, improve physical and mental performance, alleviate fatigue, and brighten mood. Their accepted roles in medicine, geriatric medicine in particular, remain in flux. Still more uncertain is the place they will have in everyday life as promoters of intellectual activity and, most problematic of all, as agents of pleasure. Our society has accepted caffeine and nicotine as stimulants. Will delivery of nicotine via cigarettes continue to decrease only to be offset by a dramatic increase in vaping-induced nicotine addiction? Will modest doses of amphetamine or methylphenidate become acceptable? Will modafinil prove to be a reasonable alternative lacking abuse liability? The only certainty is that these drugs will not fade away.

NOTES

1. Blejer-Prieto H (1965) Coca leaf and cocaine addiction—Some historical notes. *Canad Med Assoc J* 93:700–705.
2. Corning JL (1886) *Local Anesthesia in General Medicine and Surgery*. New York: D. Appleton & Company.
3. Nieman A (1860) Ueber eine neue organische Base in den Cocablattern. *Inaug. Diss.* Gottingen.
4. Mortimer WG (1901) *Peru History of Coca, "the Divine Plant" of the Incas*. New York: J.H. Vail & Co.
5. Freud S (1884) *Ueber Coca*. In English translation in S. Freud (1963) *The Coca Papers* 1–26. Vienna: Dunquin Press.
6. Liljestrand G (1967) Carl Koller and the development of local anesthesia. *Acta Physiol Scand* S299:1–30.
7. Jones E (1953) *Sigmund Freud: Life and Work*, vol. 1. London: Hogarth Press.
8. Brady KT, Lydiard RB, Malcom R, Ballenger JC (1991) Cocaine-induced psychosis. *J Clin Psychiatry* 52(12):509–512.
9. Bourke J (2010) Enjoying the high life: Drugs in history and culture. *The Lancet* 376:1817.
10. Udell GG (1972) *Opium and Narcotic Laws*. Washington, D.C.: U.S. Government Printing Office.

11. Hammond WA (1886) Cocaine and the so-called cocaine habit. *NY Med J* 12:67–69.
12. Ring FW (1887) Cocaine and its fascinations, from a personal experience. *Medical Record*, September 3.
13. Imber, G (2011) *Genius on the Edge, The Bizarre Life of Dr. William Stewart Halsted.* New York: Kaplan.
14. Cohen S (1975) *JAMA* 231(1):74–75.
15. Hyman S (2001) A 28-year-old man addicted to cocaine. *JAMA* 286(20):2586–2594.
16. Zirin D (2013) The death of Len Bias, my generation's one-person shock doctrine. *The Nation* 18 November.
17. Sheff N (2008) *TWEAK: Growing Up on Methamphetamines.* New York: Atheneum Books for Young Readers.
18. Smith P (2016) *When Meth Was Medicine: Big Pharma Amphetamine Ads from the Days of Better Living Through Chemistry.* https://www.alternet.org/drugs/when-meth-medicine-big-pharma-amphetamine-ads
19. DECODOG (2017) Stimulants, amphetamines, weight reduction drugs. http://www.decodog.com/inven/MD/md28009.jpg
20. Rasmussen N (2011) Medical science and the military: The Allies use of amphetamine during World War II. *J Interdis History* 42:205–232.
21. Bradley C (1937) Behavior of children receiving Benzedrine. *Am J Psychiatr* 94:577–582.
22. Bradley C (1950) Benzedrine and dexedrine in the treatment of children's behavior disorders. *Pediatrics* 5(1):24–37
23. Centers for Disease Control (2017) National prevalence of ADHD and treatment: New statistics for children and adolescents, 2016. https://www.cdc.gov/ncbddd/adhd/features/national-prevalence-adhd-and-treatment.html
24. Still GF (1902) Some abnormal psychical conditions in children: The Goulstonian lectures. *The Lancet* 1:1008–1012.
25. Feloni R (2013) These are the ridiculous ads Big Pharma used to convince everyone they have ADHD. *Business Insider.* https://www.businessinsider.com/adhd-medication-marketing-techniques-2013-12
26. Szalavitz M (2012) Drugging poor kids to boost grades in failing schools: One doc says yes. *New York Times*, October 10.
27. Marnell C (2017) *How to Murder Your Life: A Memoir.* London: Ebury Press.
28. Volkow ND, Swanson JM (2013) Adult attention deficit-hyperactivity disorder. *NEJM* 369:1935–1944.
29. Mayo Clinic (2018) Adult attention-deficit/hyperactivity disorder (ADHD). https://www.mayoclinic.org/diseases-conditions/adult-adhd/diagnosis-treatment/drc-20350883
30. Centers for Disease Control and Prevention (2018) Percentage of women aged 15 through 44 who filled prescriptions for ADHD, United States, 2003–2015. *Morb Mort Wkly Rep* 67(2):66–69.
31. Smith GM, Beecher HK (1959) Amphetamine sulfate and athletic performance. I. Objective effects. *JAMA* 170(5):542–557.
32. Shea J (2003) Gwynn targets amphetamines: Estimates half of position players use "greenies." *SFGate*, April 23. https://www.sfgate.com/.../Gwynn-targets-amphetamines-Estimates-half-of-26207 85.php
33. Anonymous (2008) Baseball's ADD epidemic. *USA Today*, January 17.
34. Scheindlin S (2003) Ephedra: Once a boon, now a bane. *Molecular Interventions* 3(7):358–360.

35. Holmstedt B, Liljestrand G (1963) *Readings in Pharmacology.* London: Pergamon Press.
36. Drug Enforcement Administration (2005) Combat Methamphetamine Epidemic Act of 2005. https://www.deadiversion.usdoj.gov/meth/index.html
37. Anonomous. Scourge upon scourge. *The Economist* 28: March 9, 2019.
38. Doll R, Hill AB (1952) A study of the aetiology of carcinoma of the lung. *BMJ* 2(4797):1271–1286.
39. Centers for Disease Control and Prevention (2017) Smoking and tobacco use. https://www.cdc.gov/tobacco/data_statistics/index.htm
40. Anonymous (2012) Tobacco in the USA: Smoke and mirrors. *The Lancet* 379:288.
41. Giannakoulas G, Katramados A, Melas N, Diamantopoulos I, Chimonas E (2003) Acute effects of nicotine withdrawal syndrome in pilots during flight. *Aviat Space Environ Med* 74(3):247–251.
42. Davies D (1999) Please, not wrinkles. *The Lancet* 354:264.
43. Hens G (2017) *Nicotine.* Translated by Jen Calleja. New York: Other Press.
44. Jarvik Maugh TH II (2008) UCLA pharmacologist invented the nicotine patch. *Los Angeles Times.* http://latimes.com/news/obituaries/la-me-jarvik13-2008may14,0,5794862.story
45. Miech, R, Johnston L, O'Malley PM, Patrick ME (2019) Adolescent vaping and nicotine use in 2017–2018—U.S. national estimates. *NEJM* 380(2):192–193.
46. Atik A, Harding R, De Metteo R, Kondos-devcic D, Chgeong J, Doye LW, Toicos M (2017) Caffeine for apnea of prematurity: Effects on the developing brain. *Neurotoxicol* 58:94–107.
47. Cushny AR (1913) *A Textbook of Pharmacology and Therapeutics.* Philadelphia: Lea & Febiger.
48. Fox M (2013) Richard Ben Cramer, writer of big ambitions, dies at 62. *New York Times,* October 22.
49. Anonymous (1912) The influence of caffein (*sic*) on mental and motor efficiency and on the circulation. *JAMA* 307(11)1118–1119.
50. Snyder SH, Katims JJ, Annau Z, Bruns RF, Daly JW (1981) Adenosine receptors and behavioral actions of methylxanthines. *Proc Natl Acad Sci U S A* 78(5):3260–3264.
51. Volkow ND, Wang GJ, Logan J, Alexoff D, Fowler JS, Thanos PK, Wong C, Casado V, Ferre S, Tomasi D (2015) Caffeine increases striatal dopamine D2/D3 receptor availability in the human brain. *Transl Psychiatry* e549. doi:10.1038/tp.2015.46.
52. Meredith SE, Juliano LM, Hughes JR, Griffiths RR (2013) Caffeine use disorder: A comprehensive review and research agenda. *J Caffeine Res* 3(3):114–130.
53. American Psychiatric Association (2013) *Diagnostic and Statistical Manual of Mental Disorders.* Washington, D.C.: APA.
54. Reissig CJ, Strain EC, Griffiths RR (2009) Caffeinated energy drinks—A growing problem. *Drug Alch Depend* 99:1–10.
55. Meier B (2012) Monster Energy drink cited in deaths. *New York Times,* October 22.
56. Freedman N et al. (2012) Association of coffee drinking with total and cause-specific mortality. *NEJM* 366(20):1891–1904.
57. Bastuji H, Jouvet M (1988) Successful treatment of idiopathic hypersomnia and narcolepsy with modafinil. *Prog Neuropsychopharmacol Biol Psychiatry* 12(5):695–700.
58. Volkow ND et al. (2009) Effects of modafinil on dopamine and dopamine transporters in the male human brain: Clinical implications. *JAMA* 301(11):1148–1154.

CHAPTER 5

∽∾

Depressants:
Sedative-Hypnotic-Tranquilizing Drugs

From Errant Yeast to Halcion and Its Relatives

The agents we will consider in this chapter are a disparate bunch, but they are united in that most can induce a mild state of intoxication that many of us find to be pleasant; social drinkers of ethyl alcohol are familiar with the phenomenon. The darker side of these drugs is that all can induce physical dependence with a characteristic and sometimes life-threatening withdrawal syndrome. In addition, they are often agents of addiction; alcoholism is a prime example. Further uniting these drugs is the relatively recent recognition of a common mechanism of action. Their current primary medical uses are in anesthesiology, as anticonvulsants, and in the treatment of anxiety and sleep disorders.

For many years, drugs of this class were referred to as sedative-hypnotics. Sedation implies the induction of a state of calmness, while hypnosis refers to sleep. However, with the discovery of meprobamate (Miltown), and the benzodiazepines, for example, Valium, which we will consider later, a third term was introduced. These drugs were to be called *tranquilizers* to distinguish them from earlier sedative-hypnotics. But whatever the drugs are called, the fact is that for most there is a dose-related continuum of action beginning with a state of calmness (call it tranquility, if you wish) to sleep, and, finally, for some, coma and death.

Our Love Affair with Drugs: The History, the Science, the Politics. Jerrold Winter, Oxford University Press (2020). © Jerrold Winter.
DOI: 10.1093/oso/9780190051464.001.0001

An illustration of the long-recognized connectedness of sedation, hypnosis, and anxiety was provided us by Henry Behrend. He describes his patient as

> ... a gentleman, forty years of age. ... He was of a most excitable and nervous
> temperament, and was engaged in mercantile transactions of great magnitude,
> the extent of which seemed quite to overwhelm him. ... He had lost his natural
> sleep, was harassed and fatigued during the day, and sought my opinion as to
> whether he ought not at once to withdraw from business, although the sacrifice
> entailed thereby would be very great, and he was most anxious to avoid it.[1]

Fortunately, following drug treatment, the patient was, according to Dr. Behrend, "able to sleep perfectly well, has regained spirits and confidence, and has quite abandoned the idea of his unfitness to attend to his business transactions." While we might imagine Dr. Behrend's patient to be a 21st-century denizen of The City or Wall Street, treated perhaps with Xanax or Prozac or another of the many drug options available, the year was in fact 1864 and the drug was potassium bromide, about which more will be said later in this chapter.

ANXIETY AND ITS RELIEF

Unlike stimulants such as cocaine and the amphetamines with their direct mood-elevating actions, the attractiveness of depressant drugs for humans and their physicians resides primarily in their ability to relieve anxiety, a condition familiar to all of us. Anxiety is Nature's way of keeping us moving. Much of our growth as human beings comes as we contend with anxiety-provoking situations. For many it begins with separation from our mothers and proceeds through every phase of our lives.

All agree that anxiety is a normal reaction to stress and serves a useful purpose in driving us to achieve whatever it is we wish to achieve. To erase all forms of anxiety could do great harm. Freed from the motivating force of anxiety, we might simply drop out and, regrettably, many have found that sedative-hypnotic drugs are a facilitator of that process. But when anxiety interferes with our ability to effectively interact with others and to carry out the tasks of daily life, it is a distinct handicap rather than a stimulus to action. In addition, anxiety is often a most unpleasant state. In such situations, drug treatment may be very helpful. Finally, anxiety accompanies many diseases and may interfere with effective treatment and recovery;

the example of intense anxiety resulting from a diagnosis of cancer immediately comes to mind. There was a time not long ago when those suffering from anxiety were labeled as being neurotic. The term is no longer used; instead, we suffer from *anxiety disorders*, a category housing a multitude of conditions, including panic attacks, obsessive-compulsive disorder, post-traumatic stress disorder, social phobia, and, most common of all, generalized anxiety. It has been estimated that, in any given year, 10% of the adult population of the United States experiences an anxiety disorder.[2]

DEPRESSANT DRUGS AND DEPRESSION

Before undertaking an examination of individual drugs, a clear distinction must be drawn between the terms *depression* and *depressant drugs*. In the course of a lifetime, nearly all of us experience fluctuations in mood. These episodes of sadness and joy often can be traced to readily identified events in our lives. A new job or the birth of a baby or a wedding is joyful, while the opposite affective state may be engendered by disappointment in love, the death of a friend, or financial losses. Sometimes our mood is up or down without apparent reason. When we are down, we are said to be depressed. Such fluctuations are entirely normal.

When swings in mood are extreme or unrelenting, we enter the world of psychiatry. In addition to severe anxiety, we may experience clinical depression, a mental state characterized by sadness, changes in appetite and sleep, and feelings of hopelessness. Anxiety and insomnia often accompany depression. There is loss of interest or pleasure in our normal activities. (Shakespeare's sonnet 29: "With what I most enjoy contented least.") In its most extreme form, depression is accompanied by thoughts of suicide, thoughts which may end in death.

In contrast with a mood or affective state, the *depression* of depressant drugs refers to a decrease in the level of activity of the receptors on which the drug exerts its effects. When acting on the heart, a depressant drug may decrease the rate of beating or the force of contraction. In the brain, the firing rate of neurons is decreased. In chapter 2 we saw how heroin, fentanyl, and other opioids act to decrease the activity of neurons of the medulla oblongata to slow the rate of breathing to the point where death may result. (In this respect, opiates too are depressant drugs but traditionally are separated from sedative-hypnotics on the basis of their mechanisms of action and their medical and recreational uses.)

But if depressant drugs decrease activity of the neurons of our brains, how do we explain a noisy bar on Saturday night? While it is true that depressant drugs may induce sleep, they can also act to dampen the activity of areas of the brain that normally suppress behavior. Thus, the prototypic depressant drug, ethyl alcohol, may result in a release of inhibitions and stimulation of behavior. Recall that stimulants such as the amphetamines used in the treatment of attention-deficit/hyperactivity disorder reliably result in a decrease in unproductive activity. While some may view as paradoxical the stimulation of behavior by a depressant drug or suppression of behavior by a stimulant drug, I prefer to see these as predicable consequences of the interaction of drugs with the complexities of our brains. Having said that, depressant drugs in general, while they may disinhibit behavior at modest doses, may, at higher doses, suppress the activity of regions of the brain to the point of death.

ALCOHOL: MOTHER NATURE'S GREAT DEPRESSANT

The Kingdom Fungi includes molds and yeasts. Mention a fungus infection or mold in your pantry, and you are likely to elicit an alarmed look. But it was a fungus infection by a blue-green mold called *Penicillium notatum* of a Petri dish containing *Staphylococcus aureus* in the laboratory of Sir Alexander Fleming that led ultimately to penicillin, a truly wondrous drug.[3] Several hundred million years before this, another member of the fungi family, an airborne yeast, came into contact with downed plant material and, as yeasts are wont to do, some of the plant's sugar was converted into ethyl alcohol. From fruit came wine, and from grain it was beer; mirabile dictu, the cacao plant gave us chocolate beer. Thus did humans come to possess ethyl alcohol, the first sedative-hypnotic-tranquilizing drug. Just exactly when humans harnessed these natural experiments is not known, but archaeologists have found evidence from 10,000 years ago.

Ethyl alcohol is representative of a family of organic chemicals called alcohols. However, for our purposes, it is only ethyl alcohol that is of interest as a depressant drug, and I will subsequently refer to it simply as *alcohol*. The effects of alcohol, like those of most other drugs, are dose related. Modest doses are associated with a variety of mood changes, which may include feelings of well-being, self-confidence, and talkativeness. As the dose increases, signs of sedation and motor incoordination will appear, which may then progress to sleep, coma, and, in extreme intoxication, death. Feelings of self-confidence combined with motor incoordination are major factors in the lethality of drunk driving.

Just one other alcohol is worth mentioning here: methyl alcohol or methanol. It is a component of many perfumes, cosmetic products, window cleaners, and antifreeze. Its consumption often leads to blindness and even death. An event that occurred in 2016 in Irkutsk, an impoverished city in Siberia, is illustrative. Unable to afford even the cheapest of vodka, alcoholics turned to a scented bath lotion containing methanol; more than 50 died as a result.[4]

PHYSICAL DEPENDENCE ON ALCOHOL

With the regular use of alcohol, a modest degree of tolerance will develop, accompanied by the development of physical dependence. The abstinence syndrome, which results when alcohol is denied to a physically dependent person, is first characterized by tremors, nausea, anxiety, irritability, and changes in blood pressure and heart rate. Untreated, the syndrome may progress to what has been called alcoholic epilepsy or "rum fits" in which convulsions occur. Somewhat later, delirium tremens (the DTs), may appear with agitation, insomnia, and vivid hallucinations.[5] Perhaps the most famous cinematic illustration of the DTs was provided by Don Birnam, a character in the film *The Lost Weekend*.

Although delirium tremens was not described in the medical literature until the early 1800s[6] and not produced experimentally until 1955 in former morphine addicts[7] confined to the United States Narcotic Farm described in chapter 2, the ethanol withdrawal syndrome was recognized by Hippocrates several centuries before the birth of Christ: " . . . if the patient be in the prime of life, and . . . if from drinking he has trembling hands, it may well be to announce beforehand, either delirium or convulsion."[8]

Avoidance of the ethanol withdrawal syndrome is essential. Death may result in those untreated. For the alcoholic, the method of choice to avoid withdrawal is to continue drinking. (Those who have viewed *The Lost Weekend* can recall Don Birnam's desperate searches for a source of alcohol.) In a medical setting, avoidance of withdrawal is accomplished by the use of one of the other drugs in the depressant class which exhibits cross-physical dependence with alcohol. In earlier times, a barbiturate would be used, but presently a drug of the benzodiazepine class such as Librium or Valium is the usual choice.[9]

AT LAST, A RECEPTOR FOR ALCOHOL

As ancient as is man's use of alcohol, it was only late in the 20th century that pharmacological science provided a plausible explanation for how it works in our brains. Embedded in the outer covering of our neurons is a variety of channels that control the inward and outward flow of essential chemicals, which in turn control the excitability of the neuron. One such channel is called $GABA_A$, named for *gamma*-aminobutyric acid, a neurotransmitter that acts upon the channel to suppress firing and thus maintain a normal level of excitation in the nervous system.[10] Alcohol acts at the $GABA_A$ receptor to augment this effect. I mention this bit of esoterica because it now appears that the same mechanism accounts for the effects of nearly all drugs used for anxiety and insomnia. Even propofol, the drug implicated in Michael Jackson's death, acts this way. The existence of a common mechanism of action explains how these depressant drugs can be additive or even more than additive in their effects. As one amateur pharmacologist put it: A Xanax and a beer is as good as a six-pack. (More about Xanax in a moment.) Also explicable is the phenomenon of cross-tolerance and cross-physical dependence; earlier I mentioned that a barbiturate or benzodiazepine can prevent the alcohol withdrawal syndrome. A curious and currently inexplicable observation familiar to anesthesiologists is that alcoholics typically require higher concentrations of anesthetic gases to achieve and maintain unconsciousness.[11]

THE MEDICAL USES OF ALCOHOL

During the 18th and 19th centuries, the medical literature was often the site of conflicting views regarding the therapeutic usefulness of alcohol.[12] However, despite concerns expressed about alcoholism, the consensus was that alcohol could serve as an essential source of calories and a stimulant for frail bodies. Many regarded alcohol as a panacea for acute diseases, including the much-feared yellow fever.

In 1795, New York City leased the 5-acre Bel-Vue estate located on the East River "to serve as a hospital for the accommodation and relief of such persons afflicted with contagious distempers." Instructions for a yet-to-be-named medical director were explicit: "Sherry wine, the most natural stimulus, should be given freely . . . beer, for those who are accustomed to its use, is a very valuable remedy." In his elegant tale of the hospital, David Oshinsky tells us that David Hosack, founder of the modern Bellevue Hospital, confronted with "a rash of tetanus," prescribed "wine, spirits and brandy" so the patients at least would have "a more peaceful demise."[13] In 1850s England, a patient with pneumonia, typhus, or rheumatic fever might expect to be "brandied," given 3 pints of brandy per day for several days to a month. Though many studies have suggested that alcohol in moderation is beneficial to human health, especially with respect to heart disease, few advise drinking for our health or to treat our ailments. Indeed, a massive evaluation of the global health consequences of alcohol consumption recently concluded that the ideal level of intake is no intake at all.[14]

Mention of brandy reminds us of another improvement on nature made by man. Beer, wine, and other natural ferments are limited in their maximum alcohol content to 10%–15% percent by the fact that alcohol in greater concentration inactivates yeast and shuts off the fermentation process. However, fractional distillation, a process that makes use of the fact that alcohol boils at a lower temperature than water, allows the production of alcoholic beverages with much higher alcohol content. Although crude methods of distillation date back at least a thousand years, the process came into full flower beginning in the early 18th century. This had important consequences, not the least among them that the descent from recreational drinking to alcoholism became much easier. While it is true that one can become addicted to beer or wine, alcoholism is more likely to occur with the use of rum, gin, bourbon, vodka, moonshine, or any of the other products of distillation that contain on the order of 50% alcohol (100 proof).

Soon after gin was introduced into Great Britain late in the 17th century, concern was expressed that drunkenness and criminal activity had significantly increased. In response, the Gin Act of 1751 placed heavy taxes on the sale and consumption of gin. I mention this only to draw your attention to two prints issued at the time by William Hogarth in support of the Gin Act. One is called *Beer Street*, whose inhabitants are happy and healthy. In contrast, those of *Gin Lane* are dissolute and dying.

ALCOHOLISM AS A DISEASE

Now let us consider alcoholism in somewhat greater detail. The pharmacological facts are inescapable. Taken in sufficient dose for a sufficient period, alcohol induces physical dependence of what is called the alcohol-barbiturate type. I have already described the withdrawal syndrome. More important, often accompanying this physical dependence is alcohol addiction. There arises a behavioral state of compulsive, uncontrolled alcohol craving and seeking; the alcoholic is an addict. Equally inescapable is the toll taken by alcoholism on the individual and upon society. For example, the combination of poor nutrition and the direct toxic effects of alcohol upon the liver may lead to alcoholic cirrhosis, a condition which alone takes about 20,000 lives in the United States each year. The Centers for Disease

Control and Prevention estimates that the figure for all alcohol-related deaths exceeds 100,000 per year.[15]

In 1784, Benjamin Rush, MD, psychiatrist, signer of the Declaration of Independence, and Surgeon-General of the Continental Army, published a book in which he explicitly called intemperate use of alcohol a disease and referred to it as an addiction.[16] A more explicit expansion of Rush's view was provided by Magnus Huss, a professor of medicine at the Caroline Institute in Stockholm. The year was 1852.[17] A century later, the American Medical Association, the American College of Physicians, and the American Psychiatric Association were in agreement with the view that alcoholism is a disease and a legitimate target of medical intervention. Nonetheless, from colonial times to the present, controversy has continued among scientists, physicians, and the general public as to whether alcoholism should be considered a physical disease such as diabetes or cancer, the consequence of a combination of mental, social, and physical factors, or simply a moral failing.

Alcoholics Anonymous, founded in 1935, was clear in its view: Drinking is a symptom of disease, an alcoholic has an incurable vulnerability to alcohol, and an alcoholic can never drink again. Following World War II, scientific support for this view came from E. Morton Jellinek, a biostatistician who became a leader in studies of alcoholism. In 1960, Jellinek published *The Disease Concept of Alcoholism*, in which he argued that for the alcoholic a single drink begins an inevitable process that ends in addiction.[18] This so-called loss of control became a central tenant of the disease hypothesis.

The concept of alcoholism as an incurable disease was not without its detractors. In 1988, Herbert Fingarette, an emeritus professor of philosophy at the University of California, published *Heavy Drinking: The Myth of Alcoholism as a Disease*.[19] He stated that alcoholism is merely a label that covers "a variety of social and personal problems caused by the interplay of many poorly understood physiological, psychological, social, and cultural factors." No less august a body than the US Supreme Court agreed with Fingarette. Lawyers representing two veterans had argued that their clients failed to apply for benefits in the required time frame because of their disease of alcoholism. Veterans Affairs countered that the men had engaged in willful misconduct. The Court agreed with Veterans Affairs, and benefits were denied.

I will not attempt to reconcile these differing views on the roots of alcoholism but would refer you to my comments in chapter 2 with respect to opiate addiction. I believe that they apply equally well to alcoholism. There I expressed my belief that the roots of addiction are multiple and include physical, mental, and social factors. And, as I stated in chapter 2 with respect to opiate addicts, the majority of alcoholics will benefit from treatment. The most famous non–drug approach is that of Alcoholics Anonymous. Its Twelve-Step Program emphasizes an acknowledgment of powerlessness over alcohol and an appeal to a higher power. There are countless other treatment programs, many of uneven quality, which suffer from the same defects as described in chapter 2 for opiate treatment programs. With respect to pharmacological aids to therapy, the options are limited; only three drugs are currently approved.

DRUGS AGAINST ALCOHOLISM

Shortly after World War II, a Copenhagen cocktail party led directly to disulfiram, best known by its trade name Antabuse, as a means to deter alcoholics from drinking.[20] Jens Hald and Erik Jacobsen, scientists at a Danish pharmaceutical house, had been seeking drugs to kill intestinal worms. One evening the young men became violently ill following their accustomed alcohol ration. In much the same way that Albert Hofmann traced his first LSD trip to a chemical he had been working with in his laboratory, Drs. Hald and Jacobsen intuited that one of their anti-parasite drugs, disulfiram, had altered their reaction to alcohol. Hald and Jacobsen published their findings on Christmas Day 1948 in *The Lancet*. In that same issue, their Danish colleague, Oleg Martensen-Larson, described disulfiram treatment of alcoholics in a paper titled "Treatment of Alcoholism With a Sensitizing Drug."[21]

Following the drinking of alcohol, its intoxicating effects recede as our bodies metabolize the drug. The ultimate products are carbon dioxide, water, and energy, but the first step in the process yields acetaldehyde. Disulfiram, by blocking the further conversion of acetaldehyde, allows toxic levels to accumulate. The consequences for the drinker, as experienced by Hald and Jacobsen, are dramatic and may include pulsating headache, nausea, vomiting, blurred vision, confusion, and chest pain. The alcoholic, having been warned of this effect of disulfiram, is expected to stop drinking or, if a drink is taken, to suffer the consequences. Antabuse was approved for use in the United States in 1951 and remains available today. As plausible as is the underlying rationale for the use of Antabuse, this form of aversive therapy is not acceptable to many alcoholics and dropout rates are high. Nonetheless, the drug remains a part of many treatment programs.

The second anti-alcoholism drug to be considered is already familiar to us. It is naltrexone, a close relative of naloxone (Narcan), the drug discussed in chapter 2 that is now widely distributed to rescue opiate users from impending death from overdose. These drugs act by blocking opiate receptors in the brain. By the early 1990s evidence had accumulated from animal experiments that opiate receptors might be involved in the actions of alcohol. From this there evolved the hypothesis that naltrexone might decrease the craving for alcohol. To test the hypothesis, a study was conducted in 70 alcoholics at the Philadelphia Veterans Affairs Medical Center.[22] The results indicated that naltrexone decreased both drinking and relapse to drinking. Subsequent studies have generally supported the results seen in the veterans.[23]

Naltrexone, with the trade name Revia, was approved for use in 1994 for the treatment of alcoholism. One of its shortcomings was the need for daily administration. This was addressed in 2006 with the introduction of a sustained-release form of naltrexone (Vivitrol) that is given by injection once a month.

The third drug of our triumvirate, acamprosate (Campral), has been in use in Europe since 1989 but was not approved for use in the United States until 2004. The way in which acamprosate works is uncertain, but actions at both depressant and excitatory systems in the brain seem likely. Studies of the drug in alcoholics suggest that it works about as well as does naltrexone.[24]

It has been argued that the designation of alcoholism as a disease is a convenient fiction that allows us to believe that a drug will be found to cure it. Given what we know about addiction, whether it be to cocaine, heroin, alcohol, or any of the other drugs that come to exert control over human behavior, the seeking of a curative magic bullet is likely to remain elusive. Surely, Antabuse, naltrexone, and acamprosate are not cures for alcoholism. On the other hand, they often serve as useful adjuncts to psychosocial treatment programs. (The use of drugs such as LSD and psilocybin will be discussed in chapter 7.)

SIR CHARLES LOCOCK, THE BROMIDE ION, AND EPILEPSY

As was discussed in chapter 3 regarding marijuana as therapy, epilepsy is an ancient disease with many forms and causes. Known to Hippocrates and mentioned in the Torah several centuries before the birth of Christ, epilepsy is characterized by seizures that may be accompanied by loss of consciousness. Modern neurology tells that these seizures are due to abnormal, excessive, hypersynchronous discharges from an aggregate of central nervous system neurons. Simpler explanations prevailed in earlier times; epilepsy was routinely attributed to possession by Satan. Strenuous exorcisms with sometimes fatal outcomes were performed. Epileptics might be regarded as insane and confined to lunatic asylums.

The Royal Medical and Chirurgical Society met in London on May 11, 1857. Following a presentation on epilepsy by a member of the group, Sir Charles Locock, president of the Society and obstetrician to Queen Victoria, commented on how he had used potassium bromide to treat "hysterical epilepsy," fits which occurred in conjunction with menstruation and which he attributed to "sexual excitement."[25] Many at that time believed that masturbation was a cause of epilepsy, and Sir Charles had been told that potassium bromide decreases sexual drive. Observing that the excitement in his patients was calmed, Locock began to treat nonmenstrual epilepsy, again with good results. The first effective anti-epileptic drug had been discovered.

The calming and anti-anxiety effects of the bromide ion in conditions other than epilepsy did not go unnoticed. At the outset of this chapter, I related to you the story of Henry Behrend's sleepless and anxious patient and his successful treatment with potassium bromide in 1864. As an alternative to opium, Behrend was of the opinion that "its importance cannot well be overrated." Within a few years, hundreds of patent medicines containing bromide appeared. I will describe just one: *Dr. Miles Nervine*, a mixture of three bromide salts.

First introduced in the early 1880s, recommendations for use of Nervine included, in addition to epilepsy, insomnia, pain, heart conditions, the ravages of tobacco smoking, and, of course, anxiety, usually referred to as "nervousness." Women were singled out for especially aggressive marketing. One advertisement had the following text.

> Nervous women are the first to lose their youth and charm . . . when your nerves get beyond control, your beauty vanishes . . . any woman who is nervous, blue, or irritable, soon loses her attractiveness and begins to look old . . . (Nervine) promptly sooths and calms you . . .[26]

In 1938, nonprescription sales of bromide products in the United States were second only to those of aspirin. But something peculiar was going on; in that same year, it was recommended that all psychiatric patients be tested for bromide intoxication. Despite the fact that bromides share with alcohol the ability to calm the anxious, induce sleep, and produce physical dependence and addiction, they hold a surprise as well. It is a form of intoxication called *bromism*.

The signs and symptoms of bromism include confusion, irritability, memory loss, headache, loss of appetite, emotional instability, fatigue, disorientation, and depression. Tremors, weakness, and inability to walk are common. In the elderly, these effects may be interpreted as the onset of dementia and, in those of all ages, may be confused with a psychiatric disorder.[27]

As an anti-epileptic, bromides were displaced by drugs we will discuss in the next section, but it was bromism which prompted the Food and Drug Administration to ban all over-the-counter sleep aids containing bromides. Bromide intoxication today is uncommon but not nonexistent. In 2009, an infant girl, just 22 days of age, was brought to the emergency room of a New York City hospital because of excessive sleepiness and a loss of appetite. For the previous 12 days her parents had been giving her Cordial de Monell, a product intended to treat colic.[28] Produced in the Dominican Republic and popular among the Dominican community in New York, its active ingredient is potassium bromide. The case prompted a warning from the New York City health department.

CHLORAL HYDRATE: THE MICKEY FINN

In the years following the discovery of the anti-epileptic and anxiety-relieving properties of the bromide ion, nearly a dozen other drugs with somewhat similar properties were found. I will mention just one: chloral hydrate. Still in use today as an anesthetic agent, chloral hydrate gained fame as the *Mickey Finn*. Named for a Chicago saloon keeper of the late 19th century, the drug would surreptitiously be slipped into the drink of a patron so that he might more easily be robbed; an added benefit was that the victim would be left with little memory of the event. More recently, the depressant actions of chloral hydrate have found use in combination with those of morphine and secobarbital in a lethal cocktail for use in states such as Oregon and California that permit physician-assisted dying.[29],[30]

Chloral hydrate is the ancestor of today's date-rape drugs such as GHB and Rohypnol, which will be discussed shortly. But it was another drug, barbital, that changed the face of sedation and hypnosis and displaced potassium bromide as an anti-epileptic agent.

THE CHILDREN OF ST. BARBARA

In chapter 1, I told you that the marriage of organic chemistry and physiology resulted in the birth of pharmacology as a medical science. It was in Germany in particular that organic chemistry flourished. Two of its most distinguished contributors were Adolf von Baeyer and his student, Emil Fischer. Later, student and mentor would each receive the Nobel Prize in Chemistry, Fischer in 1902, von Baeyer in 1905. It was von Baeyer who in 1864 synthesized a chemical to be called *barbituric* acid. The story of its naming is contested, but the one I find most appealing is that *uric* refers to urea, a waste product found in urine, and *barbit* to St. Barbara, patron saint of the artillerymen with whom von Baeyer and his colleagues celebrated their discovery at a local tavern. Barbituric acid has no sedative properties, but hundreds of related chemicals would subsequently be synthesized and their pharmacological properties explored.

The first to enter medical practice from the family now called barbiturates was barbital in 1903. It was in that year that Fischer and Joseph von Mering, a physician, described in the German medical literature what they called a new class of hypnotics.[31] It was to be sold under the trade name *Veronal*. Whether the name was derived from *verus*, the Latin word for "truth," as in the first true hypnotic, or from Verona, the Italian city where von Mering is said to have learned by telegram of its synthesis by Fischer, is a matter of dispute. Worldwide use for the treatment of insomnia and anxiety soon followed for Veronal and its many relatives, which included phenobarbital in 1912 and amobarbital in 1923. The latter would gain fame as a supposed truth serum, though its efficacy in that regard has never been firmly established. In the 1930s there came secobarbital, thiopental, and hexobarbital. (In the classic film *Grand Hotel*, the troubled ballerina Grusinskaya famously says, "Not even the Veronal can help me sleep.")

Over the course of the first four decades of the 20th century, barbiturates gained great popularity as the mainstay of the treatment of anxiety and insomnia. The medical profession regarded barbiturates as both highly useful and relatively safe, although deaths from overdose, whether accidental or with suicidal intent, were reported with some regularity. By 1950, a billion doses a year were being taken.

Recognition of barbiturate-induced physical dependence and addiction was slow in coming, but this was not for lack of warning signs. A paper published in 1925 from the Los Angeles General Hospital reported 61 cases of what was called "Veronal poisoning."[32] In it, the authors referred to addiction in many of the users. The physicians' attitude toward their patients was clear: ". . . an unstable and inferior part of society . . . the diagnosis of constitutional psychopathic inferiority was made in a number of instances . . ." This assessment of the barbiturate addict brings to mind the words of Lawrence Kolb, whom we met in chapter 2, in describing the majority of opiate addicts as psychopaths. Recall that Dr. Kolb was the chief medical officer of the federal narcotic prison in Lexington, Kentucky. Today, condemnation of addicts in such terms is not a part of a 21st-century approach to treatment. But it was in Lexington that the issue of physical dependence on barbiturates was definitively settled.[33]

BARBITURATE PHYSICAL DEPENDENCE

In 1950, despite their extensive use, barbiturates were not believed to induce physical dependence. The prisoners of the Lexington narcotic farm provided ready subjects to test that belief. In an initial report, four of five men suffered convulsions following abrupt withdrawal of secobarbital. Subsequently those five plus fourteen others were treated with one of two dosing regimens for a period of 45 days. The severity of the physical dependence thus induced was dose related in that three quarters of those given the higher dose convulsed upon withdrawal but only 10% following the lower dose. The issue of physical dependence on barbiturates was settled.

The signs and symptoms of barbiturate withdrawal are strikingly similar to those we saw earlier for alcohol. Indeed, we now refer to physical dependence of the alcohol/depressant type. Following chronic use, abrupt termination of a barbiturate is followed by a progressive decrease in intoxication for 6 to 15 hours. The withdrawal syndrome then begins with anxiety, nervousness, tremor of hands and face, progressive weakness, loss of appetite, nausea, vomiting, and insomnia. This may then progress to convulsions, hallucinations, delirium, and, in some instances, death.[34] Indeed, in 1975, the deaths of Drs. Stewart and Cyril Marcus, attending physicians at New York Hospital, were attributed by the Medical Examiner to barbiturate withdrawal. The brothers had been long-time users of barbiturates, but little of the drug was present in their body tissues at the time of death. It was speculated that they might have been attempting to end their physical dependence.[35]

DR. HAUPTMAN'S EPILEPTIC PATIENTS

Today, newer drugs have eclipsed but not entirely replaced the barbiturates for the treatment of anxiety and insomnia. However, phenobarbital remains an essential anti-epileptic drug, especially for young children. The story of the discovery of the use of phenobarbital for epilepsy is an interesting one.[36] In 1912, Alfred Hauptmann was a 31-year-old physician in Freiburg, Germany, who, as a junior staff member, was assigned sleeping quarters above a ward for epileptic patients. Disturbed by the noise of their seizures during the night, he gave the patients phenobarbital as a sedative but noticed as well that their seizures were diminished. The drug was soon marketed with the trade name Luminal. In 2017, 105 years after discovery of its anti-epileptic properties, it retains its place on the World Health Organization's *Essential Drug List*. Though nonmedical use of barbiturates peaked in the United States in the 1970s, the drugs remain popular for their pleasurable effects, to reduce anxiety, and as a moderator of the effects of stimulant drugs such as cocaine. (As a result of the Nuremberg Laws of 1935, Dr. Hauptmann, a Jew, was made to give up his university professorship. After a brief stay at Dachau, the infamous Nazi concentration camp, he was able to make his way to the United States, where he remained for the rest of his life.)

DEATH AND DIGNITY

One other current use of barbiturates is worthy of mention: reliable and painless induction of death. "Death and Dignity" was the title of an article published in the *New England Journal of Medicine* on March 7, 1991.[37] The author was Timothy Quill, MD, an attending physician at the Genesee Hospital in Rochester, New York. In it, Dr. Quill told how he had assisted the suicide by barbiturate overdose of Diane, his 45-year-old patient. Dr. Quill's article was a remarkable admission not the least because in New York State a person convicted of aiding in a suicide is liable to 5–15 years imprisonment. (A grand jury in Rochester subsequently declined to indict him.)

In November 1997, the State of Oregon approved the Death With Dignity Act. The Act allows terminally ill adult Oregonians to obtain from their physician a prescription for a lethal dose of a medication, usually pentobarbital or secobarbital. The physician does not administer the drug. Instead, the patient fills the prescription and self-administers the drug at a place and time of his or her choosing. In Oregon, more than nine in ten die at home. By 2018, similar laws had been passed in Washington, Vermont, Montana, Colorado, Hawaii, California, and the District of Columbia. It is ironic that in a country where it is estimated that several hundred tons of barbiturates are manufactured each year, the price of prescription barbiturates has increased to the point where alternative lethal medications are being considered. A high-potency opiate such as fentanyl, a drug implicated in many unintended overdose deaths, is being considered, and earlier I mentioned the use of chloral hydrate for this purpose.

MILTOWN: THE FIRST TRANQUILIZER

Frank Berger took his medical degree in 1937 at the University of Prague, and he began work in infectious disease. However, his life changed abruptly with the German occupation of Czechoslovakia 2 years later. Berger was, like Alfred Hauptman, the discoverer of the anti-epileptic effects of barbiturates, a Jew, and thus a nonentity in Nazi eyes. Making his way to a government laboratory in England, he studied a drug called mephenesin. When injected into animals, mephenesin produced a somnolent state which Berger would later call *tranquilization*. Mephenesin entered medical practice as a muscle relaxant but was soon observed as well to produce in humans a relaxed state bordering on euphoria.

In 1949, having moved to the United States 2 years earlier, Berger joined Carter-Wallace Laboratories, a small pharmaceutical house in New Jersey then best known for a 19th-century patent medicine called Carter's Little Liver Pills, recommended for headache and various gastrointestinal problems. By this time Berger's interests had become focused on the treatment of anxiety and the discovery of drugs which might treat it. He regarded anxiety as a disease and believed that its relief would add to "human happiness, human achievement, and the dignity of man." A series of drugs was synthesized and tested in animals for tranquilizing effects. The most active of the group was meprobamate; a movie was created showing its calming effect in otherwise vicious monkeys. A study in humans soon followed, and meprobamate entered the marketplace in 1955 with the names Miltown and Equanil. A new era in the treatment of anxiety and insomnia had dawned.[38]

With the recognition that barbiturates produce tolerance, physical dependence, and addiction similar to alcohol, the term *sedative* become anathema. For marketing purposes, meprobamate was to be called a *tranquilizer*. To distinguish it from antipsychotic drugs such as chlorpromazine (Thorazine), meprobamate was termed a *minor tranquilizer*; antipsychotic drugs were *major tranquilizers*. The attachment to these drugs of a common term, tranquilizer, is unfortunate in that the implication is that these are similar drugs differing only in intensity of effects. Much inappropriate prescribing has resulted, including the prescription of antipsychotics for simple anxiety. But, for advertisers, tranquilizer is a wonderful word. Who, after all, would not wish to be tranquil?

In *A History of Psychiatry*, Edward Shorter's superb book on the subject, we are told that demand for meprobamate in the form of Miltown and Equanil was by 1957 "far greater than for any drug ever marketed in the United States."[39] Furthermore, in contrast with the barbiturates, meprobamate was safe; in 1956, Frank Berger could rightfully claim that all attempts at suicide with the drug had been unsuccessful. It was touted as treatment for alcoholics, smokers, and opiate addicts. But there were other reports, more ominous yet predictable from what was already known of sedative-hypnotic drugs. In the decade following its introduction, a withdrawal syndrome similar to that of the barbiturates was reported, and instances of addiction were noted. Between 1962 and 1976, meprobamate accounted for 6.5% of psychoactive drug admissions to Massachusetts General Hospital. Nonetheless, meprobamate was a quantum improvement over the barbiturates for the treatment of anxiety.

A NEW ERA: THE BENZODIAZEPINES

The reign of meprobamate did not long go unchallenged. With the huge commercial success of Milton and Equanil, the pharmaceutical industry set its synthetic chemists the goal of finding something comparable or even superior. The first to succeed was Hoffmann-La Roche, a Swiss multinational company with a major research facility in Nutley, New Jersey.

In 1940, a Polish chemist named Leo Sternbach began work in the Roche laboratories in Basel. Because Sternbach was Jewish and with Germany just a few miles away, the company wisely transferred him to Nutley the following year. Many drugs were synthesized and tested in animals; none seemed promising until what Sternbach called the last of the series, chlordiazepoxide.[40] Like meprobamate before it, chlordiazepoxide had a taming effect in monkeys and, following only minimal testing in humans, it was introduced to the market in 1960 with the name Librium. Three years later, Sternbach and Roche followed up with the second of a series in the family called benzodiazepines. This was diazepam with the trade name Valium.

The commercial success of Librium was both immediate and spectacular. Advertisements were universal in their appeal. Women were the most frequent target with the drugs recommended to relieve anxiety induced by, among other things, babies and toddlers underfoot, unpaid bills, thinning hair, absent husbands, and simple boredom with an unfulfilled life. Men and children were not ignored. An ad that resonates with me suggests

Valium to treat the "tension that can ruin the life of men dominated by women." Accompanying the picture of a big yellow school bus and an obviously frightened little girl was the promise that Librium eases the anxieties of childhood.[41] By 1978, sales of Valium reached $1 billion, and it was the most widely prescribed drug in the world.

The benzodiazepine family now includes many other familiar names. Among them are Versed (midazolam), Xanax (alprazolam), Dalmane (flurazepam), Ativan (lorazepam), Restoril (temazepam), Rohypnol (flunitrazepam), and Halcion (triazolam). Standing marginally apart is a group of "nonbenzodiazepine" drugs used largely for insomnia. Best known are Ambien (zolpidem), Sonata (zaleplon), and Lunesta (eszopiclone). I say "standing marginally apart" because, though they chemically are not benzodiazepines, they act, as do alcohol, meprobamate, and the benzodiazepines, at $GABA_A$ receptors. Hence, we should not expect their benefits and risks to be significantly different. Zolpidem is also marketed as Intermezzo, to be taken by insomniacs who awaken in the middle of the night.

BENZODIAZEPINE, PHYSICAL DEPENDENCE, AND OTHER HAZARDS

Soon after Librium went on sale, it was reported that the drug produces physical dependence.[42] The withdrawal syndrome closely mimics that of alcohol and the barbiturates, and seizures are not uncommon. Reports of addiction were soon to follow. The similarities of the benzodiazepine and alcohol withdrawal syndromes are such that Librium and others of its family remain essential tools in treating withdrawal in alcoholics; that is, they exhibit cross-physical dependence. Despite the early recognition in the medical community of physical dependence and addiction to the benzodiazepines, the phenomena did not gain wide public attention until 1979 with the publication of Barbara Gordon's book *I'm Dancing as Fast as I Can*, a vivid description of her withdrawal from Valium.[43]

A major virtue of the benzodiazepines is that, compared with the barbiturates, it is much more difficult to kill yourself with an overdose. However, their effects in combination with alcohol and opiates are less certain, and there is the suspicion that they may contribute to a fatal outcome. Anecdotal evidence for this possibility comes from public disclosure of autopsy results following the death of celebrities. For example, benzodiazepines were among the multiple drugs found in Heath Ledger, Michael Jackson, Corey Heim, and Whitney Houston.

While anxiety and its treatment with benzodiazepines may run throughout our lives, the aging brain, and especially the demented brain, is particularly susceptible to the adverse effects of these drugs. Nonetheless, benzodiazepines continue to be used frequently in the elderly and, in addition to the possibility of confusion and physical dependence, are a major contributor to fall-related injuries. For this reason, some have gone so far as to advise that all benzodiazepines be avoided in the elderly. In addition, subtle signs of benzodiazepine withdrawal can be misinterpreted as a worsening of dementia leading to further inappropriate drug treatment.

Despite the relative safety of the benzodiazepines in causing death when taken in excess, several epidemiological studies have found a peculiar increase in the risk of death in elderly persons treated with acceptable doses of these drugs. It has been difficult to pinpoint an exact cause for this fact, but a report published in 2013 suggests a possible contributor. Eneanya Obiora and his colleagues examined the association between the use of benzodiazepines and the occurrence of pneumonia. Use of benzodiazepines increased the risk of pneumonia by almost 50%. In the nearly 5,000 patients studied, the risk of death from the disease was increased by 20% to 30%.[44]

THE PECULIAR EFFECTS OF HALCION

From the time that Librium came to market to the present day, various members of the benzodiazepine family have been associated with what have been called "paradoxical reactions": depression, paranoia, memory loss, irritability, increased anxiety, aggression, suicidal thoughts, and even outright violence. Halcion (triazolam), a drug which became the most frequently prescribed sleeping pill in the world, is of particular interest.

In 1979, a Dutch psychiatrist described some alarming effects in his patients treated with Halcion.[45] These included aggression, hallucinations, and severe suicidal tendencies. Three years later, the Upjohn Company (now Pharmacia & Upjohn) received approval to market the drug in the United States. Later it would be alleged that the company failed to disclose to the Food and Drug Administration "paranoid events" observed in inmates at Michigan's Jackson State Prison in whom the drug had been tested. In June 1988, a Utah woman named Ilo Grundberg killed her 83-year-old mother by firing eight bullets into her head. Ms. Grundberg had been taking Halcion for about a year. She was charged with murder but was acquitted on the grounds of an "involuntary intoxication." Following a lawsuit by Ms. Grundberg, Upjohn did not admit liability but provided her a multi-million-dollar settlement.[46]

With respect to Halcion and suicide, two American writers have provided vivid descriptions. William Styron, author of *Darkness Visible: A Memoir of* Madness,[47] was suffering from insomnia brought on by anxiety concerning an impending surgical procedure. A prescription for Halcion was provided. Subsequently Styron was "totally consumed by thoughts of suicide . . . thinking only of walking out into the ocean and being engulfed by the waves."[48] Philip Roth tells a similar tale in his novel *Operation Shylock*.[49] He was taking Halcion for insomnia following minor knee surgery. In Roth's words, "I thought about killing myself all the time." Alas, multiple anecdotes, even by distinguished authors, do not add up to scientific data. At this time, the Food and Drug Administration says only this: "In primarily depressed patients, the worsening of depression, including suicidal thinking, has been reported . . . " Triazolam was banned in the United Kingdom in 1991.

GHB AND THE DRUGS OF DATE RAPE

Anesthesiology is the only branch of medicine in which drug-induced loss of memory, amnesia, is considered a good thing. Specifically, anterograde amnesia, loss of memory for events in the recent past, is a desirable property of a benzodiazepine such as midazolam (Versed). Often given in combination with an opiate, midazolam decreases recall and in doing so enhances patient tolerance and acceptance of surgical and diagnostic procedures. Unfortunately, there is a darker side to anterograde amnesia, and it is another benzodiazepine, Rohypnol (flunitrazepam), which is its poster child.

It has been estimated that 17% of American women and 3% of men will be the victim of rape or attempted rape at some time during their lifetime. Fully 75% of these assaults will be at the hands of an acquaintance or date, hence the term "date rape." Although Rohypnol is not approved for use in the United States, it is readily purchased online and is a popular club drug. When surreptitiously dissolved in a convenient drink, Rohypnol is colorless, odorless, and tasteless. Particularly when taken in combination with alcohol, the drug will produce sedation, euphoria, and disinhibition. Most important, there will be anterograde amnesia. Many persons who have been violated will have no firm memory of what transpired. In such instances, it is now advised that a urine test for the presence of Rohypnol in potential victims be conducted.

The final drug we will consider in this chapter is an odd but interesting one. It goes by the initials GHB. Earlier I mentioned the presence in our brains of a chemical called *gamma*-aminobutyric acid, which functions to depress neuronal activity. Pharmacologists have long thought that if GABA could be used as a drug, we would have a natural alternative to alcohol, barbiturates, and benzodiazepines. Unfortunately, GABA does not enter the brain following oral administration; this is due to what is called the blood–brain barrier, which blocks some drugs while allowing others such as THC and nicotine to pass with ease. But it turns out that a simple chemical alteration of GABA yields *gamma*-hydroxybutyric acid or GHB, which readily enters the brain and, as predicted, has rather unique sedative properties.

GHB, which can refer to both the acidic form and to its sodium salt, was first isolated by Henri Laborit, a French military surgeon whose lasting fame rests on his identification of the therapeutic properties of Thorazine (chlorpromazine), the first effective antipsychotic agent. In 1960, Laborit reported the first use of GHB as an anesthetic agent.[50] In the nearly six decades since, GHB has been found useful in the treatment a variety of conditions calling for a sedative. Thus, it has been advocated for use in controlling the withdrawal syndrome to alcohol and as a maintenance agent for alcoholics.[51]

Presently, in the United States, the sodium salt under the trade name Xyrem is approved only for use in narcolepsy, a condition characterized by excessive daytime sleepiness sometimes accompanied by cataplexy, a sudden loss of muscle power. It may seem odd that a sedative would have value in treating narcolepsy. By way of explanation, it has been suggested that perhaps, by improving normal nighttime sleep, GHB diminishes daytime sleep. Alternatively, GHB has been noted to have some stimulant properties. In 2010, Jazz Pharmaceuticals, the US manufacturer of Xyrem, sought approval for its use in fibromyalgia, a much more common condition than narcolepsy, hence representing a much greater market potential. Approval was denied by a committee of the Food and Drug Administration which expressed concern about possible diversion and abuse of the drug.

GHB might have remained merely a pharmacological curiosity confined to use in narcoleptics had it not been for the report in 1977 by Japanese pharmacologists that GHB stimulates the release of human growth hormone in male volunteers.[52] In the presence of deficiency of growth hormone, children will not reach normal height, and treatment with the hormone is highly valued and effective. More controversial is the use of the hormone in healthy children destined to be short in stature.

In addition to its medical use, growth hormone is much valued by athletes of all kinds and bodybuilders and others interested in increased muscle mass and strength. Its reputation is much like that of the anabolic steroids. And, like the steroids, use of growth hormone is banned by many athletic federations, including the International Olympic Committee. Fans of baseball will recall the controversy surrounding allegations of use by Roger Clemens and Barry Bonds—allegations said to be a factor in their nonelection to the National Baseball Hall of Fame. In 2013, major league baseball began random tests of its players for the presence of excess growth hormone.

Largely based on the ability of GHB to increase levels of growth hormone, the drug soon became widely promoted and widely used in the bodybuilding and athletic communities. Concurrent with this illicit use was the recognition of GHB's properties as a sedative-hypnotic with the ability to induce euphoria, disinhibition, and anterograde amnesia; in the early 1990s it became a popular club drug. At the same time, GHB took its place along with Rohypnol as an agent of seduction and assault. Political response took the form of the Hillary Farias and Samantha Reid Date-Rape Drug Prohibition Act of 2000. Samantha and Hillary died following the use of GHB at age 15 and 17, respectively.[53] The Act placed GHB in Schedule 1 and thus deemed it as having a high liability for abuse and no accepted medical use.

NOTES

1. Behrend H (1864) Action of the bromide of potassium in inducing sleep. *The Lancet* I:607–608.
2. Comer JS, Blanco C, Hasin DS, Liu SM, Grant BF, Turner JB, Olson M (2011) Health-related quality of life across the anxiety disorders. *J Clin Psychiatry* 71(1):43–50.
3. Fleming A (1929) On the antibacterial action of cultures of a Penicillium with special reference to their use in the isolation of *B. influenzae*. *Brit J Exp Path* 10:226–236.
4. Nechepurenko I (2016) In Russia, dozens die after drinking alcohol substitute. *New York Times*, December 19.
5. Mello NK, Mendelson JH (1977) Clinical aspects of alcohol dependence. In *Drug Addiction I*, WR Martin, Ed. Berlin: Springer-Verlag.
6. Pearson SB (1813) Observations on brain fever; delirium tremens. *Edinb Med Surg* 9:326–332.
7. Isbell H, Fraser HF, Wikler A, Belleville RE, Eisenman (1955) Experimental study of the etiology of rum fits and delirium tremens. *Q J Stud Alcohol* 16(1):1–33.
8. Zillborg G, Henry GW (1941) *A History of Medical Psychology*. New York: W.W. Norton & Co.

9. Santos C, Olmedo RE (2017) Sedative-hypnotic drug withdrawal syndrome: Recognition and treatment. *Emerg Med Pract* 19(3):1–20.

10. Brohan J, Goudra BG (2017) The role of GABA receptor agonists in anesthesia and sedation. *CNS Drugs.* 31(10):845–856.

11. Han YH (1969) Why do alcoholics require more anesthesia? *Anesthesiology* 30:341–342.

12. Warner JH (1980) Physiological theory and therapeutic explanation in the 1860's: The British debate on the medical use of alcohol. *Bull Hist Med* 54:236–257.

13. Oshinsky D (2017) *Bellevue: Three Centuries of Medicine and Mayhem at America's Most Storied Hospital.* New York: Doubleday.

14. Burton R, Sheron N (2018) No level of alcohol consumption improves health. *The Lancet* 392(10152):987–988.

15. Centers for Disease Control and Prevention (2018) Fact sheets—Alcohol use and your health. https://www.cdc.gov/alcohol/fact-sheets/alcohol-use.htm

16. Rush B (1811) *An Inquiry Into the Effects of Ardent Spirits upon the Human Body and Mind, With an Account of the Means of Preventing, and of the Remedies for Curing Them*, 6th edition. New York: Cornelius Davis.

17. Huss M (1852) *Chronische Alkoholskrankheit oder Alkoholismus Chrnoicus.* Translated into German from the Swedish. Originally published 1849. Leipzig: CE Fritze.

18. Jellinek EM (1960) *The Disease Concept of Alcoholism.* Highland Park, NJ: Hillhouse.

19. Fingarette F (1988) *Heavy Drinking, The Myth of Alcoholism as a Disease.* Berkeley: University of California Press.

20. Hald J, Jacobsen E (1948) A drug sensitizing the organism to ethyl alcohol. *The Lancet* 2:1001–1004.

21. Martensen-Larsen O (1948) Treatment of alcoholism with a sensitizing drug. *The Lancet* 2:1004–1007.

22. Volpicelli JR, Alterman AI, Hayashida M, O'Brien CP (1992) Naltrexone in the treatment of alcohol dependence. *Arch Gen Psychiatry* 49:876–880.

23. Soyka M, Rosner S (2008) Opioid antagonists for pharmacological treatment of alcohol dependence—A critical review. *Curr Drug Abuse Rev* 1(3):280–291.

24. Kalk NJ, Lingford-Hughes AR (2014) The clinical pharmacology of acamprosate. *Br J Clin Pharmacol* 77(2):315–323.

25. Locock C (1857) in discussion, Sieveking EH, Analysis of 52 cases of epilepsy by the author. *The Lancet* 1:524–528.

26. Pinterest (2018) Vintage ads for Dr. Miles Nervine liquid and tablets. https://www.pinterest.com/pin/304626362265365476/

27. Carney MWP (1971) Five cases of bromism. *The Lancet* 2:523–524.

28. Lugassy DM, Nelson LS (2009) Case files of the Medical Toxicology Fellowship at the New York City Poison Control: Bromism: Forgotten but not gone. *J Med Toxicol* 5(3):151–157.

29. Harman SM, Magnus D (2017) Early experience with California End of Life Option Act. *JAMA Internal Med* 177(7):907–908.

30. Aleccia J (2016) Death with Dignity doctors create new medication. *Seattle Times*, April 4.

31. Fischer E, Mering J von (1903) Ueber eine neue Klasse von Schlafmitteln. *Ther d Gegenw* 44:97–101.

32. Leake WH, Ware ER (1925) Barbital (Veronal) poisoning. *JAMA* 84(6):434–436.

33. Fraser HF, Wikler A, Essig CF, Isbell H (1958) Degree of physical dependence induced by secobarbital or pentobarbital. *JAMA* 166(2):126–129.

34. Fraser HF, Jasinski DR (1977) The assessment of the abuse potentiality of sedative/hypnotics (depressants). In *Drug Addiction I*, WR Martin, Ed. Berlin: Springer-Verlag.

35. Marcus brothers deaths Rensberger B (1975) Death of 2 doctors poses a fitness issue. *New York Times*, August 15.

36. Yasiry Z, Shorvon SD (2012) How phenobarbital revolutionized epilepsy therapy: The story of phenobarbital therapy in epilepsy in the last 100 years. *Epilepsia* 53(s8):26–39.

37. Quill, TE (1991) Death and dignity: A case of individualized decision making. *NEJM* 324:691–694.

38. Shorter E (1997) *A History of Psychiatry*. New York: John Wiley & Sons.

39. Sternbach LH (1983) The benzodiazepine story. *J Psychoactive Drugs* 15(1–2):15–17.

40. Sternbach LH (1983) The benzodiazepine story. *J Psychoactive Drugs* 15(1–2):15–17.

41. World Benzodiazepine Awareness Day (2018) w-bad.org/vintage/ads

42. Anonymous (1977) Physical dependence on benzodiazepines? *Drug Ther Bull* 15(22):85–86.

43. Gordon B (1979) *I'm Dancing as Fast as I Can*. New York: Harper & Row.

44. Obiora E et al. (2013) The impact of benzodiazepines on occurrence of pneumonia. *Thorax* 68:163–170.

45. Van der Kroef C (1990) Reactions to triazolam. *The Lancet* 2:526.

46. Dyer C (1991) Triazolam settlement. *BMJ* 303:433–434.

47. Styron W (1990) *Darkness Visible: A Memoir of Madness*. New York: Random House.

48. Styron W (1993) Prozac days, Halcion nights. *The Nation*, January 4.

49. Roth P (1993) *Operation Shylock*. New York: Simon & Schuster.

50. Laborit H, Jouany JM, Gerard J, Fabiani F (1960) Generalites concernant l'etude experimentale de l'emploi du *gamma*-hydroxybutyrate de Na. *Aggressiologie* 1:397–406.

51. Addolorato G, Cibin M, Caprista E, Beghe F, Gessa G-L, Stefanini GF, Gasbrrini G (1998) Maintaining abstinence from alcohol with *gamma*-hydroxybutyric acid. *The Lancet* 351:38.

52. Takahara J, Yunoki S, Yakushiji W, Yamauchi J, Yamane Y (1977) Stimulatory effects of gamma-hydroxybutyric acid on growth hormone and prolactin release in humans. *J Clin Endocrinol Metab* 44(5):1014–1017.

53. H.R. 2130—106th Congress. Hillory J. Farias and Samantha Reid Date-Rape Drug Prohibition Act of 2000. https://www.govtrack.us/congress/bills/106/hr2130>

CHAPTER 6

⚭

Dissociative Anesthetics

Angel Dust to Special K to Ketamine Clinics

We will consider just two drugs in this chapter. They are phencyclidine and ketamine. Both are widely used as anesthetic agents, ketamine in humans and phencyclidine in animals. The acronym for phencyclidine that we will use, PCP, comes from its chemical name 1-(1-PhenylCyclohexyl)-Piperidine. In addition to their medical use, both ketamine and PCP have gained roles as recreational drugs or, as others would put it, drugs of abuse. While sharing some of the properties of the depressant drugs we met in the preceding chapter, PCP and ketamine are pharmacologically and therapeutically unique.

PCP BECOMES ANGEL DUST

On March 26, 1956, V. Harold Maddox, a chemist working at the research laboratories of Parke, Davis & Company in Detroit, synthesized a novel compound later to be called phencyclidine. PCP was submitted in the autumn of that year for testing in animals. Pigeons, mice, rats, Guinea pigs, rabbits, dogs, cats, and monkeys all had their turn. Depending on the dose employed and the species in which it was tested, the effects ranged from excitement and stimulation to taming and quieting. Analgesia, that is, absence of pain without loss of consciousness, and anesthesia were common

Our Love Affair with Drugs: The History, the Science, the Politics. Jerrold Winter, Oxford University Press (2020). © Jerrold Winter.
DOI: 10.1093/oso/9780190051464.001.0001

but, unlike the depressant drugs we met in the previous chapter, the anesthesia was not accompanied by depression of breathing.[1]

Studies in human subjects began in May 1957 at the Department of Anesthesiology of the Detroit Receiving Hospital. By this time, PCP had been given the trade name Sernyl. The drug initially was administered to seven volunteers. As had previously been noted in animals, there was no suppression of breathing or disturbance of cardiac rhythm, highly desirable qualities in an anesthetic agent. The investigators then moved on to 64 patients ranging in age from 18 to 78, 47 of whom were women, who were to undergo various surgical procedures, including breast biopsy, dilation and curettage, skin grafts, hysterectomy, and hernia repair.[2]

Immediately after the intravenous administration of PCP, there was what the anesthesiologists called "a profound state of analgesia" permitting surgical incision and, in many cases, completion of the operation without the use of other drugs. Most remarkably, the patients were in what one investigator called "a trance-like state with eyes open, not appearing to be asleep or anesthetized, but rather disconnected from the surroundings." However, in 13 of the group, adverse effects were seen. These ranged from mild excitement to a manic state to convulsive movements. It was concluded that, as had been observed in animals, PCP can act as both a depressant and a stimulant.

Postoperatively, most patients were happy and even euphoric, and none had any memory of their surgical procedure. However, a significant number experienced what were called "emergence reactions." Some became excited, agitated, and unmanageable, a clear danger in a hospital setting. However, some observers would note the resemblance of emergence reactions to the catatonic stupor of schizophrenia: immobile, mute, and unresponsive, yet fully conscious. Based on these effects, the United States Army Chemical Warfare Laboratories studied the possible use of PCP as an incapacitating agent.

The emergence reactions were sufficient to doom the chances of PCP ever gaining approval for use as an anesthetic agent in humans. Nonetheless, aspects of the PCP experience would prove attractive to those who seek altered states of consciousness; some described pleasant feelings of numbness, weightlessness, and floating; others spoke of what can best described as an out-of-body experience, the sense that one is an observer of one's physical self.

Illicit use of PCP began to appear on the West Coast of the United States in 1968 and, soon thereafter, PCP joined the ranks of "club drugs" favored by the young. It went by various names, perhaps the most attractive being "Angel Dust." By the mid-1970s, use of PCP had reached what some called epidemic proportions. Political response took the form of the Psychotropic Substances Act of 1978, which tightened controls over the sale of a precursor to PCP synthesis.[3]

In the decades following the 1978 Act, PCP's popularity as a recreational drug has waxed and waned. The most recent data of which I am aware indicate that some 6 million Americans have experienced the drug at least once. A sign that the drug has not lost its appeal is a 2013 report that emergency room visits due to PCP showed a four-fold increase between 2005 and 2011.[4] Currently, the drug is often found as an additive to marijuana products. Fortunately, deaths following the use of PCP are relatively uncommon, and these are usually attributable to irrational behavior under the influence of the drug rather than to direct toxic effects.[5] I noted the amnesia that accompanies its use.

KETAMINE: THE TAMING OF PCP

PCP remains today widely used in veterinary medicine, but a tamer version would be required for use in human patients. The specific goal was to reduce the intensity and duration of the emergence reactions. At the Parke, Davis & Company laboratories, a program of chemical synthesis resulted in more than 300 variations of PCP, all of which were tested in animals. The most promising of these candidates, given the label CI-581, was able to produce in monkeys anesthesia superior to that of PCP. On October 3, 1964, the first patient received CI-581. Ketalar was the name given to CI-581.

In 1965, Edward Domino and his colleagues at the University of Michigan Medical Center described the effects of ketamine in 20 prison inmates. In their report, they coined the term *dissociative anesthesia*.[6] It referred to the peculiar state of unconsciousness produced by ketamine in which the subject is unresponsive to pain and in a trance-like state, not appearing to be asleep or anesthetized, but rather disconnected from the surroundings. It appeared that there was a dissociation between sensory inputs, including pain, and the usual responses to them; in effect, the prisoners experienced sensory isolation. In 1970, ketamine was approved by the Food and Drug Administration (FDA) for human use. Today there are many who advocate sensory isolation by nondrug means such as a darkened, soundproof room or a flotation tank in order to reduce anxiety and pain or to facilitate meditation and to foster creativity. Thus, it is not difficult to imagine that the ease of ketamine-induced sensory isolation might prove attractive to adventurous individuals.

In each of the preceding chapters, the phenomena of drug tolerance, physical dependence, and addiction have been noted. Here again, ketamine and PCP are unique in that only minimal tolerance and physical dependence have been shown, and addiction to their use is not often seen. This is not to say that there are no adverse consequences following chronic use. These include impairment of memory, delusional states, and depression.[7]

Recognition of the adverse effects of illicit use of *Special K, as* ketamine came to be called, has led to efforts to ban its use entirely. At the March 2015 meeting in Vienna of the Commission on Narcotic Drugs, it was proposed, for the fourth time since 2006, that ketamine be placed in the same category as LSD and other psychotropic drugs, a move that would make ketamine unavailable for medical applications. In December of that year, the World Health Organization (WHO) rejected the proposal; ketamine would remain on WHO's Essential Medicines List. Dr. Marie-Paule Kieny, the Director General for Health Systems at WHO, said this: "The medical benefits of ketamine far outweigh potential harm from recreational use. Controlling ketamine internationally could limit access to essential and emergency surgery, which would constitute a public health crisis in countries where no affordable alternatives exist."[8]

KETAMINE AND DEPRESSION

A new and currently unfinished chapter in the story of ketamine opened on December 10, 1997, at the annual meeting of the American College of Neuropsychopharmacology in Kona, Hawaii. It took the form of a talk by investigators from the Yale University School of Medicine entitled "The Effects of Ketamine in Major Depression."[9] Based on studies in animals suggestive of an antidepressant effect,[10] seven depressed patients had been given intravenous infusions of ketamine. All exhibited significant improvement in their depressive symptoms as measured by a standard rating scale. More remarkable was that depression lifted within days.

Today's favorite antidepressant drug is Prozac (fluoxetine), a member of the family of drugs called selective serotonin reuptake inhibitors (SSRIs). Serotonin is a neurotransmitter believed to be involved in a variety of essential functions, including appetite for food and sex, as well as having a role in depression. However, SSRIs are slow to act; several weeks may be required for discernable antidepressant effects to appear. This is a significant drawback in that suicide is an ever-present danger. Indeed, there may be an increase in suicidal behavior in the early days of treatment with an SSRI. Only electroconvulsive therapy works quickly; for this reason it is often the treatment of choice in patients at immediate risk of suicide. A drug able to act rapidly to lift depression would represent a highly significant advance.

Perhaps because of the reputation of ketamine as a potential drug of abuse or the need for intravenous infusion, few paid much attention to the 1997 oral report or to publication of the results 3 years later. That all changed in August 2006 with a study by a group working at the National Institute of Mental Health (NIMH).[11] Eighteen patients unresponsive to previous drug therapy were treated with ketamine. All exhibited relief of their depression within 2 hours and the beneficial effect remained significant for a week.

Aided in no small measure by the public relations arm of the National Institutes of Health, the ketamine findings were widely reported. The *Washington Post*: "Government workers announced that they have had striking success in treating depression in a matter of hours." The *Boston Globe*: "Ketamine has the power to lift stubborn depression within hours." *Nature*: "This could be the key to understanding depression." *The Economist*: "Ketamine has opened up a new line of attack on a horrible illness." Neely Tucker of the *Washington Post* waxed poetic: "Depression is blown away like a petal on a passing breeze." A former director of NIMH would say that "ketamine, given intravenously, might be the most important breakthrough in antidepressant treatment in decades." Enthusiasm in the popular press did not recede. The cover story of *Time* magazine for August 7, 2017, described ketamine, somewhat belatedly, as "a surprising new drug."

In discussing the many claims made for medical marijuana in chapter 3, I mentioned the Cochrane Group. Many regard their reviews as the gold standard for the evaluation of treatment for medical conditions of all kinds. The Cochrane review of ketamine in 2015 was based on 25 studies of depression. Their assessment was guarded: "We found limited evidence for ketamine's efficacy over placebo at times up to one week . . . the effects were less certain at two weeks post-treatment. . . . Despite the promising nature of these preliminary results, our confidence in the evidence was limited by risk of bias and the small number of participants."[12] In 2015, the Research Task Force on Novel Treatments, an arm of the American Psychiatric Association (APA), concluded that given the "fleeting nature" of benefit and its "potential for abuse and neurotoxicity," ketamine's use "warrants caution." The APA group emphasized the current absence of information regarding the possible neurotoxic effects of long-term use of ketamine. Expressing concern about the abuse liability of ketamine, they suggested that "diversion of prescribed ketamine for illicit use could rival, or even exceed, problems currently encountered with prescription opiates . . . "[13]

Entrepreneurial physicians are not to be deterred by an APA Task Force or by a Cochrane review. You may recall that any drug approved by the FDA for any condition may be prescribed "off-label" by any physician for any other condition. The example given in chapter 4 was the use of stimulant drugs, approved for the treatment of ADHD, to improve school performance in non-ADHD children. Thus, perfectly legal *ketamine clinics* have now sprung up across the United States; as of 2017, 34 states and the District of Columbia had at least one each; California led with six.[14] At these clinics, one can receive a regular intravenous infusion of ketamine; some recommend once a week. Treatment does not come cheap. In New York City, your *Special K* was priced in 2017 at $575 for the initial infusion and $475 per visit thereafter. As well as treating depression, many of these clinics recommend ketamine for posttraumatic stress disorder, chronic pain, and anxiety. As a treatment unapproved by the FDA, any insurance you may have is unlikely to be of help.

An alternative to off-label intravenous infusion of ketamine was provided by the FDA in March 2019 with the approval of a nasal spray called Spravato. You may recall that in chapter 4 we spoke of the mirror images of amphetamine; these were referred to as the *d*- and *l*- isomers. Spravato is esketamine, one of the two isomers of ketamine. It has been shown to act more quickly than a mixture of the *S*- and *R*- isomers. Taken in combination with a standard antidepressant drug, Spravato will not come cheaply; Janssen Pharmaceuticals estimates a course of treatment will cost somewhere between $4,720 and $6,785. But, as an approved FDA-approved drug, insurance may be of some help. The drug will be available only in a certified medical office and cannot be taken home.

PCP: A MODEL FOR PSYCHOSIS?

Shortly after PCP was first given to a human subject in 1957, the drug came into the hands of Elliott Luby, a psychiatrist at the Wayne State University College of Medicine in Detroit. Dr. Luby was struck by the similarity of PCP's effects to some aspects of psychosis. Indeed, the title of his first PCP publication was "Study of a New Schizophrenomimetic Drug."[15]

The hope was that an understanding of PCP's actions might lead to insight into the biological bases of psychosis and, in turn, to the discovery of more effective drug treatments. Similar hopes for depression accompanied the discovery, four decades later, of the antidepressant effects of ketamine. Today, those hopes remain largely unfulfilled but, as Alexander Pope expressed it, hope springs eternal in the human breast. (When Dr. Luby conducted his studies, companies such as Parke, Davis & Company freely distributed their drugs to interested parties. Times have changed.)

THE PCP RECEPTOR

Before leaving these fascinating drugs, I want to say just a bit more about how they might act. For pharmacologists, the holy grail is often the discovery of the receptor or receptors upon which a drug exerts its initial effects. In chapter 2, we saw how isolation of the opiate receptors led not only to a clearer understanding of how opiates work as drugs but also to the identification of previously unrecognized natural chemicals, the endorphins, and the physiological system upon which they work. A similar story was told in chapter 3 regarding marijuana, THC, and the cannabinoid system.

In 1979, a PCP receptor was identified in rat brain, and it was shown that both PCP and ketamine act upon it.[16] In the years that followed, considerable controversy surrounded the nature of the PCP receptor and how it might be linked to the myriad of effects observed with the dissociative anesthetics. Current thinking is that the PCP receptor is located within an ion channel called the NMDA receptor; thus, we have a receptor upon a receptor; nature is indeed complicated. The natural occupants of the NMDA receptor are glutamate and glycine. Their effects are blocked by PCP and ketamine; for this reason, PCP and ketamine are called NMDA antagonists.

It was in 1990 that Ramon Trullas and Phil Skolnick hypothesized that "pathways subserved by the NMDA subtype of glutamate receptors are involved in the pathophysiology of affective disorders . . ."[17] Their study used mice as subjects and examined, not PCP or ketamine, but, instead, other members of what was now a family of NMDA antagonists. Nonetheless, their hypothesis led directly to the test of ketamine as an antidepressant in human subjects and to today's ketamine clinics.

The pharmaceutical industry has shown great interest in discovering NMDA antagonists that are ketamine-like in terms of relieving depression but devoid of ketamine's less desirable adverse effects. None of the drugs so far tested has met those criteria. These negative results have led some to suggest that ketamine may be acting in some as yet undiscovered way that does not involve NMDA receptors. The brain is indeed a complicated organ.

NOTES

1. Maddox VH, Godefroi, Parcell RF (1965) The synthesis of phencyclidine and other 1-arylcyclohexylamines. *J Med Chem* 230–235.
2. Greifenstein FE, Yoshitaki J, DeVault M, Gajewski JE (1958) 1-aryl cyclo hexyl amine for anesthesia. *Anesthesia Analgesia* 37(5):283–294.
3. S. 2399—95th Congress (1978) Psychotropic Substances Act. https://www.govtrack.us/congress/bills/95/s2399>
4. Bush DM (2013) *Emergency Department Visits Involving Phencyclidine (PCP): The CBHSQ Report.* Rockville, MD: Substance Abuse and Mental Health Services Administration, November 12.
5. Dominici P, Kopec K, Manur R, Khalid A Damiron K, Rowden (2015) Phencyclidine intoxication Case Series Study. *J Med Toxicol* 11(3):321–325.6.
6. Domino EF, Chodoff P, Corssen G (1965) Pharmacological effects of CI-581, a new dissociative anesthetic. *Clin Pharmacol Ther* 6(3):279–291.7.
7. Dillon P, Copeland J, Jansen K (2003) Patterns of use and harms associated with non-medical ketamine use. *Drug Alcohol Depend* 69:23–28.8.
8. Kieny M-P (2015) WHO recommends against international control of ketamine. www.who.int/medicines/access/controlled-substances/recommends_against_ick/en/
9. Cappiello A, Charney D, Berman R, Anand A, Miller H, Oren D (1997) The effects of ketamine in major depression. Abstr. American College of Neuropsychopharmacology, 36th Annual Meeting.
10. Trullas R, Skolnick P (1990) Functional antagonists at the NMDA receptor complex exhibit antidepressant actions. *Eur J Pharmacol* 185:1–10.
11. Zarate CA, Singh JB, Carlson PJ et al. (2006) A randomized trial of an NMDA antagonist in treatment-resistant depression. *Arch Gen Psychiatry* 63:856–864.
12. Coddy C, Amit BH, McCloud TL, Rendell JM, Furakawa TA, McShane R, Hawton K, Cipriani A (2015) Ketamine and other glutamate receptor modulators for depression in adults. *Cochrane Data Base Syst Rev* 23(9):CDO11612.
13. Newport DJ, Carpenter LL, McDonald WM, Potash JB, Tohen M, Nemeroff CB (2015) Ketamine and other NMDA antagonists: Early clinical trials and possible mechanisms of depression. *Am J Psychiatry* 172(10):950–966.
14. Ketamine Advocacy Network—Provider Directory (2017) of U.S. providers of ketamine therapy for depression, bipolar, PTSD, and other mood disorders. http://ketamineadvocacynetwork.org/provider-directory/
15. Luby ED, Cohen BD, Rosenbaum G, Gottlieb JS, Kelley R (1959) Study of a new schizophrenic drug—Sernyl. *Arch Neurol Psychiatry* 81:363–369.
16. Vincent JP, Kartalovski B, Geneste P, Kamenka JM, Lazdunski M (1979) Interaction of phencyclidine ("angel dust") with a specific receptor in rat brain membranes. *Proc Natl Acad Sci USA* 76(9):4678–4682.
17. Trullas R, Skolnick P (1990) Functional antagonists at the NMDA receptor complex exhibit antidepressant actions. *Eur J Pharmacol* 185:1–10.

CHAPTER 7

cνɔ

Hallucinogens

*Magic Mushrooms, Ayahuasca, Mescal Buttons,
and Dr. Hofmann's Problem Child*

There are about 400,000 species of plants in this world. Only a small
fraction, perhaps 100 in number, contain hallucinogenic chemicals.[1]
Nearly a century ago, Lewis Lewin, professor of pharmacology at the
University of Berlin, in speaking of drugs he called *phantasticants*, said
"The passionate desire which . . . leads man to flee from the monotony of
daily life . . . has made him discover strange substances (which) have been
integral to human evolution both societal and cultural for thousands of
years."[2]

An unusual problem presents itself to me in writing about these
drugs: They straddle the worlds of science and mysticism. The Encyclopedia
Britannica defines *mysticism* as the practice of religious ecstasies (religious
experiences during alternate states of consciousness), together with whatever ideologies, ethics, rites, myths, legends, and magic may be related to
them. Science I am comfortable with; mysticism not so much. Yet in our ex-
ploration of the agents found in this chapter, we will encounter many persons speaking of drug-induced mystical experiences. I have attempted to
get around my unease by first providing the history and the pharmacology
of these agents and then touching only lightly on mysticism, allowing
readers to draw their own conclusions.

Our Love Affair with Drugs: The History, the Science, the Politics. Jerrold Winter, Oxford University
Press (2020). © Jerrold Winter.
DOI: 10.1093/oso/9780190051464.001.0001

HALLUCINOGEN OR PSYCHEDELIC: THE CLASSICS

What shall we call these chemicals? *Hallucinogen,* a substance that induces perception of objects with no reality, is the term most commonly encountered and the one that I have settled on for the title of this chapter. However, it comes with a caveat. Albert Hofmann, the discoverer of LSD, our prototypic hallucinogen, has pointed out that a true hallucination has the force of reality, but the effects of LSD only rarely include this feature. Two additional terms that we will find useful are *psychotomimetic* and *psychedelic.* We have already considered the former, an ability to mimic psychosis, in our discussion of amphetamine-induced paranoid psychosis in chapter 4 and the effects of phencyclidine in chapter 6. A psychedelic was defined in 1957 by Humphrey Osmond, inventor of the word, as a drug like LSD "which enriches the mind and enlarges the vision."[3] *Psychedelic* together with *entheogen* (revealing the God within) are terms which come too close to mysticism for my comfort, but we find them used today by serious investigators, some of whom we shall meet later in this chapter.

I have made no attempt to provide an encyclopedic account of hallucinogens. For example, there will be no discussion of *Amanita muscaria* (fly agaric), an intoxicating mushroom which originated in Siberia, the belladonna alkaloids which are delirium-inducing anti-cholinergic drugs, or any of the other plant-derived chemicals sometimes identified as hallucinogens. Instead, we will confine ourselves to what are regarded as the classical hallucinogens. These are mescaline, lysergic acid diethylamide (LSD; the German word for acid is *sauer*), N,N-dimethyltryptamine (DMT), and psilocybin. These drugs are united in the similarities of the syndromes they induce and, we now believe, by a common mechanism of action involving brain receptors for 5-hydroxytryptamine (5-HT, serotonin), a neurotransmitter.[4,5]

A CACTUS CALLED PEYOTE

Our story begins with a small spineless cactus called peyote. It goes by the formal names *Lophophora williamsii* and *Anhalonium lewinii*.[6] It is an ancient plant; archeologists have evidence of its use in religious ceremonies thousands of years ago by the nomadic Chichimecs in the land that would become Mexico. The Spanish conquistadors who arrived in the 16th century were not pleased with what they regarded as a pagan ritual, and they made efforts to eradicate its use. Ironically, it was a Franciscan missionary,

Bernardino de Sahagun, who wrote most extensively of the plants of the region and the herbal medicines made from them. As for peyote, Sahagun believed it to be a part of witchcraft; its users "see visions of terrifying sights like the devil and were able to prophesy the future."[7] Despite the efforts of the Spaniards, the peyote religion continued to thrive in Mexico and by the end of the 19th century had spread among the Indian peoples of the American Southwest. (Confusion arises because peyote is sometimes referred to as mescal or mezcal. This happens also to be the name of a fermented alcoholic drink made from *agave*, the century plant of Mexico. Tequila is a form of mescal made exclusively from the blue agave.)

Peyote was brought to the attention of the international medical community by an article which appeared in the *British Medical Journal* on December 5, 1896. The author was Silas Weir Mitchell, a prominent Philadelphia physician. Its title was "The Effects of *Anhalonium lewinii* (The Mescal Button)."[8] A year earlier, Dr. Mitchell had presented the paper to the American Neurological Society. Mitchell described his multiple personal experiences with peyote in generally glowing terms. He wrote that "The display which for an enchanted two hours followed was such as I find it hopeless to describe in language which shall convey to others the beauty and splendor of what I saw." Mitchell did not regard his experience as what we might now call psychedelic but instead that what he had experienced were "glorified memories." He did acknowledge possible value in psychiatry as a means "to release a mob of verbal memories" but otherwise could foresee "no obvious therapeutic uses."

Despite Mitchell's pessimistic opinion as to the therapeutic value of peyote, it had been added 50 years earlier to the Mexican compendium of drugs and, in February 1889, Parke, Davis, & Company, the Detroit-based pharmaceutical house that we met in chapter 6, listed "tincture of Anhalonium lewinii" in its catalogue. The tincture was recommended as a general tonic, especially for ailments of the heart. No mention was made of hallucinations. As for recreational use, Havelock Ellis, better known for his writings on sexual matters, was inspired by Mitchell to sample peyote. He described his experience in a note to the medical profession in 1897[9] and, the next year, in an article for the general public entitled *Mescal: A New Artificial Paradise*.[10] Ellis suggested that ". . . there is every likelihood that mescal will become popular. It certainly has a great future before it with those who cultivate the vision-breeding drugs." Mitchell was not so sure: ". . . the side-effects are so pronounced that they considerably spoil the appreciation of the beautiful visual images."

THE SECRET OF PEYOTE: MESCALINE

As I mentioned in chapter 2 in describing the isolation of morphine from opium, pharmacologists are never satisfied with complex natural materials but instead seek out the pure chemicals which mediate their effects. Thus, in 1888, Lewis Lewin, the German pharmacologist with whom I opened this chapter, obtained mescal buttons, the dried, disk-shaped tops of the peyote cactus, from Parke, Davis, & Company. Lewin set out to determine the chemical constituents of the buttons, but little progress was made until the task was turned over to Arthur Heffter, a Berlin colleague. Heffter, with both medical training and superb laboratory skills, proceeded to isolate five pure chemicals from the plant material. The chemicals were alkaloids, nitrogen-containing organic bases usually found in plants. Morphine and caffeine are examples of alkaloids that we encountered in earlier chapters.

In a series of self-experiments, Heffter first established that the effects of peyote were completely mimicked by the five alkaloids in combination. He then sampled each of the five in isolation. Just one, given the name *mescaline*, produced the hallucinogenic effects of peyote. Describing his experiment on November 23, 1897, Heffter wrote the following.

> . . . the following visual images occur. At first there are violet and green spots which are not well defined, then come images of carpet patterns, ribbed vaulting, etc. From time to time single dots with the brilliant colors float across the field of vision. . . . Later on, landscapes, halls, architectural scenes (e.g., pillars decorated with flowers) also appear. . . . Nausea and dizziness are at times very distressing . . .[11]

The origin of the remarkable effects of peyote had been revealed. Following the determination of the structure of mescaline and its synthesis in 1919, humans had for the first time a pure chemical able reliably to induce hallucinations. In the years that followed, many scientific investigations of the drug took place. Some sought to exploit its value as a therapeutic agent; more about that later. Others pursued its promise as a psychotomimetic which might offer clues as to the chemical origins of psychosis. But it was Aldous Huxley, a British intellectual, who was most influential in bringing mescaline to the attention of the general public.

MESCALINE AND *THE DOORS OF PERCEPTION*

Huxley was introduced to mescaline in California in May 1953 by Humphrey Osmond, a British psychiatrist then working in Canada. As noted earlier, it was Osmond who coined the term *psychedelic*. Huxley's experiences with the drug were described in his 1954 book, *The Doors of Perception*.[12] The title chosen was a phrase taken from William Blake's 1793 poem "The Marriage of Heaven and Hell."

> If the doors of perception were cleansed every thing would appear to man as it is, Infinite. For man has closed himself up, till he sees all things thro' narrow chinks of his cavern.

Huxley believed that "Most men and women lead lives at the worse so painful, at best so monotonous, poor and limited that the urge to escape, the longing to transcend themselves if only for a few moments, is and always has been one of the principal appetites of the soul." Unfortunately, in Huxley's view, many turn to alcohol or opiates or cocaine or marijuana or any of the other mind-altering drugs available to us to satisfy these appetites. As an alternative, he envisioned "a new drug which will relieve and console our suffering species" without doing harm. Huxley did not believe that mescaline was that ideal drug partly because of its long duration of action but more important because a few would find in it not heaven but hell in the form of adverse effects, including perhaps a kind of psychosis. Nonetheless, he thought mescaline a step in the right direction.

PEYOTE AS SACRAMENT

The discovery of mescaline did not mark the end of the use of peyote. Most prominent among its advocates were members of the Native American Church (NAC). The NAC was led in the 1880s in Oklahoma by Quanah Parker, son of Peta Nocona, a Comanche chief. His surname was that of his mother, Cynthia Anne Parker, who had been kidnapped at the age of 9 and adopted by the Comanche tribe.[13] Under Parker, the NAC adopted both Christian and Native American elements, including the ceremonial use of peyote. But the way forward was not easy. The NAC was the subject of repeated legal action seeking prohibition of any use of peyote, which was, in the view of the plaintiffs, a dangerous drug.

In 1978, The American Indian Religious Freedom Act was passed in order to preserve the culture of our indigenous peoples, including Eskimos,

Aleut, Native Hawaiians, and American Indians. A portion of the act addressed "their inherent right of freedom to believe, express, and exercise (their) traditional religions . . . and the freedom to worship through ceremonials and traditional rites." Peyote was not mentioned by name, but some believed that its religious use was protected by the Act. This was not the case. In 1990, the Supreme Court of the United States ruled that the First Amendment does not protect Indians who use peyote in religious ceremonies. But legislative relief was to come in 1994 in the form of amendments to the Religious Freedom Act. This time the use of peyote was addressed explicitly: " . . . the use, possession, or transportation of peyote by an Indian for bona fide traditional ceremonial purposes in connection with the practice of a traditional Indian religion is lawful, and shall not be prohibited by the United States or any State." Those considering conversion to the Native American Church as a shortcut to legal use of peyote will be disappointed. It remains a Schedule I drug and its use, even within the confines of the NAC, is limited to those able to document that they are at least one quarter American Indian.

ALBERT HOFMANN AND HIS *PROBLEM CHILD*

Albert Hofmann was born in Baden, Switzerland, on January 11, 1906.[14] At the age of 19, he began his studies at the University of Zurich in the laboratory of Professor Paul Karrer, a distinguished scientist who in 1939 would receive the Nobel Prize in Chemistry. Following Hofmann's completion of his doctoral studies in April 1929, Karrer, who was aware of his young student's limited finances, suggested that he "Go out quickly and earn money." The place to do that, Karrer believed, was at the Sandoz Pharmaceutical Company, located just 50 miles away in Basel. A letter from Karrer addressed to Arthur Stoll, head of the pharmaceutical research division at Sandoz, noted that Hofmann was "extraordinarily capable." Hofmann began work at Sandoz on May 1, 1929. His early years at Sandoz were concerned with developing drugs which might prove useful in treating heart disease, but, in 1936, he began to explore the chemistry of ergot alkaloids.

Ergot is a fungus that grows on the grains of rye and other grasses. When bread made from flour contaminated with the fungus is eaten, a disease called *ergotism* results. During the middle ages, European plagues of ergotism were common, especially where rye breads were a staple. Two types are recognized, *ergotism gangrenous* and *ergotism convulsivus*. In southern France, a religious order was founded in 1093 to care for the victims of ergotism. The order chose St. Anthony as their patron, and ergotism came to be called *St. Anthony's fire*, in recognition of the intense heat felt in a limb prior to the onset of gangrene. As its name implies, *ergotism convulsivus* is characterized by convulsions, but, relevant to our present story, hallucinations may occur as well.

As fearsome as is the disease of ergotism, it may surprise us to learn that ergot extract has been a part of therapeutics for many centuries as a means both to speed up birth by inducing uterine contractions and to control bleeding following childbirth. But it was not until 1918 that Arthur Stoll at Sandoz discovered ergotamine, the first ergot alkaloid to be isolated. Sandoz marketed the drug in 1921 with the trade name Gynergen. Today, ergotamine's ability to constrict blood vessels of the brain finds its primary application in the treatment of migraine.

When Hofmann began his work with the ergot alkaloids in 1935, it already was known that the basic component of many was lysergic acid, a highly unstable chemical. An important early contribution by Hofmann was to devise chemical means to stabilize lysergic acid. Using this method, a series of lysergic acid derivatives was created. Number 25 in the series, designated LSD-25, was synthesized on November 16, 1938, and submitted for testing in animals.[15] The results were not sufficiently impressive to warrant further development as a heart stimulant or uterotonic. LSD-25 was ignored at Sandoz for the next 5 years.

Based upon what Hofmann would later characterize as a "strange premonition," he decided on April 16, 1943, in the midst of World War II, to resynthesize LSD-25. The story of what happened next is best told in his own words.

> Last Friday, 16 April, I was forced to stop my laboratory work in the middle of the afternoon and go home, as I was overcome by a peculiar restlessness associated with mild dizziness. Having reached home, I lay down and sank into a kind of delirium which was not unpleasant and which was characterized by extreme activity of the imagination. As I lay in a dazed condition with my eyes closed (I experienced daylight as disagreeably bright), there surged in upon me an uninterrupted stream of fantastic images of extraordinary vividness and accompanied by an intense, kaleidoscope-like play of colors. The condition gradually passed off after about two hours.[16]

Hofmann, as the good scientist that he was, "suspected some connection between these peculiar phenomena and the substance, LSD, with which I had been working." To test this possibility, on the following Monday he dissolved 250 micrograms of LSD in water and drank it. The time was 4:20 p.m. Forty minutes later, he noticed "a slight dizziness, unrest, difficulty in concentration, visual disturbances and a marked desire to laugh." His notes end at that point. Later he would recall the following.

> I asked my laboratory assistant to accompany me home as I believed that my condition would be a repetition of the disturbance of the previous Friday. While we were still cycling home, however, it became clear that the symptoms were more marked than the first time. I had great difficulty in speaking coherently, my field of vision swayed before me, and objects appeared distorted like images in curved mirrors. I had the impression of being unable to move from the spot, although my assistant told me afterwards that we had cycled at a good pace . . .[17]

Upon arriving at home, a physician was called but upon examination he found that other than a "rather weak pulse" there were no notable signs or symptoms. Hofmann's mental state was another matter.

> All my efforts of will seemed in vain; I could not stop the disintegration of the exterior world and the dissolution of my ego. A demon had invaded me and taken possession of my body, my senses, and my soul. A terrible fear that I had lost my mind grabbed me. I had entered another world, a different dimension, a different time.[18]

By 10:30 p.m., the frightening effects of the drug were diminished, and he began to have "feelings of happiness and thankfulness."

> When I closed my eyes, an unending series of colorful, very realistic and fantastic images surged in upon me. A remarkable feature was the manner in which all acoustic perceptions (e.g., the noise of a passing car) were transformed into optical effects, every sound causing a corresponding colored hallucination, constantly changing in shape and color like pictures in a kaleidoscope.[19]

After a good night's sleep, Hofmann felt "completely fit, though slightly tired."

Hofmann's companion on his now famous bicycle ride was Suzie Ramstein, his 21-year-old laboratory assistant. Two months later, Ms. Ramstein, under Hofmann's supervision, took 100 micrograms of LSD and experienced what she called "a good experience," one she would repeat on two other occasions.[20] Others sampling the drug at Sandoz included Hofmann's superiors, Arthur Stoll and Ernst Rothlin, head of the Pharmacology Department. They were struck by the potency of the drug; Hofmann's initial dose of 250 micrograms was now seen as an overdose;

80 micrograms (that is about three millionths of an ounce) worked quite nicely for Stoll and Rothlin thus making LSD several thousand times more potent than mescaline.

LSD AND PSYCHIATRY

Following the experiences of Hofmann and his colleagues, experiments were undertaken with LSD in 16 normal volunteers and 6 schizophrenic patients at the psychiatric clinic of the University of Zurich. The investigator was Werner Stoll, son of Arthur Stoll. In 1947, the junior Stoll brought LSD to the attention of the medical world in the *Swiss Archives of Neurology and Psychiatry*. The article was titled "Lysergsäure-diäthylämid, ein Phantastikum aus der Mutterkorngruppe" (Lysergic acid diethylamide, a phantasticum from the ergot group).[21] Werner Stoll added an account of his personal experience with LSD, thus becoming the first psychiatrist to experience its effects; many of his profession were to follow him. The world would never again be the same.

Sandoz gave LSD the trade name *Delysid* and, beginning in 1947, and continuing for two decades, freely distributed the drug to any interested professionals. (In 1967, I received my first supply of LSD from Sandoz in response to a simple letter of request.) In providing LSD, two uses were suggested. The first was as an aid to psychotherapy, particularly that directed at anxiety and obsessive-compulsive disorders. The second was to permit psychiatrists, by self-administration of LSD, to gain a better appreciation of what their psychotic patients were experiencing. It soon became a common practice for clinical psychologists, psychotherapists, and psychiatrists in training to experience the effects of LSD on one or more occasions.

AYAHUASCA AND RELIGION

Somewhere on the continent now called South America, at a time before history was written, a person, perhaps a witch doctor, discovered how to make a tea possessed of wondrous properties. By combining parts of two plants, later given the names *Banisteriopsis caapi* and *Psychotria viridis*,[22] a potion was prepared which found use in religious, healing, and ceremonial activities. As news of this brew spread, it was given a variety of names; *ayahuasca* is the one we will use.

Many contemporary accounts of intoxication with ayahuasca have been provided. I will quote from that of Victoria Gill, a science reporter for the BBC, who experienced ayahuasca in Brazil in 2005.

> Ayahuasca is both the most beautiful drug I have experienced and the most putrid-tasting potion I've ever imbibed. . . . I became oblivious to all save the living dream inside my head. . . . With each trip, I entered a different universe: the first one bright and primary colored; the second a dark and carnal underground; the third, a 30th century heaven, gleaming with neon features . . . my creative life was thrown into context, my place in the world revealed and my history explained.[23]

Ms. Gill also mentions that many users experience intense nausea and vomiting prior to the onset of hallucinations.

Despite attempts by colonial conquerors, their missionaries, and the governments that followed them to stamp out the use of ayahuasca in South America, its use has prevailed to this day. Brazil provides perhaps the best example of its resilience. Beginning in the late 1800s, organized religions began to form around the sacramental use of ayahuasca. Combining Christianity with Amazonian tribal beliefs, churches such as *Santo Daime* and *Uniao do Vegetal* (*UDV*; union of the plants) flourished. Largely due to the efforts of *UDV*, the Brazilian government in 1987 sanctioned the use of ayahuasca, which to that time had been a banned drug, in religious ceremonies. (Members of the *UDV* regard nausea, vomiting, and diarrhea accompanying the use of ayahuasca as signs of purification of the soul.)

In the United States, seizure of ayahuasca from a branch of the *UDV* in Santa Fe, New Mexico, led to a legal case that eventually reached the Supreme Court of the United States. On February 21, 2006, Chief Justice John Roberts issued a unanimous decision in favor of the church. Later, a similar tale played out for the Ashland, Oregon, branch of *Santo Daime*, but this time it was a local judge, with the Supreme Court decision to guide him, who allowed the importation of ayahuasca for use by the church.

Today, despite its continued illegality outside of religious use, ayahuasca groups meet regularly in New York, Los Angeles, and other cities around the country. It seems that ayahuasca has become the darling of Wall Street, Silicon Valley, and parts in between. A group in California promises that we will be able to "understand the secrets of the universe." For those who are not members of the *UDV* or *Santo Daime* and who may be concerned about legal issues, ayahuasca tours similar to that taken by Victoria Gill are available.

DMT: THE SECRET OF AYAHUASCA

Now let us turn to the chemistry of ayahuasca. Although South American and European botanists would begin to sort out the plant origins of ayahuasca beginning in the 1850s, a century would pass before the hallucinogenic substances contained in them would be identified.

In the early 1950s, Stephen Szara, a Budapest psychiatrist, read of the effects of LSD and mescaline and wondered if their study might provide the key to unlocking the cause of mental illness in which perceptual disorders and hallucinations play a role.[24] After reading Huxley's *The Doors of Perception*, Szara decided in 1955 to experience mescaline for himself. Finding the effects of the drug to be less impressive than had been described by Huxley, he turned to LSD. As I previously noted, Sandoz had been providing the drug to any interested investigators around the world. However, Szara's application for LSD was denied, perhaps because Hungary was then under the control of the Soviet Union. Undeterred, Szara recalled that *N,N*-dimethyltryptamine (DMT) had that same year been found in *Cohoba*, a South American snuff powder purported to be hallucinogenic.[25] But no one had ever tested the activity of DMT in humans. Szara himself would fill that gap in our knowledge.

Initial experiments were disappointing. Dr. Szara took increasing doses of DMT by mouth but observed no hallucinogenic effects. He then tried intramuscular injection of the drug. Following a modest dose, he experienced visual sensations that reminded him of descriptions he had read of the effects of LSD and mescaline. He then doubled the dose; the results were remarkable.

> . . . optical illusions, pseudo-hallucinations, and later, real hallucinations appeared. The hallucinations consisted of moving, brilliantly colored oriental motifs, and later I saw wonderful scenes altering rapidly. The faces of the people seemed to be masks. My emotional state was elevated sometimes up to euphoria. . . . After 45 minutes to 1 hour the symptoms disappeared and I was able to describe what had happened.

Szara confirmed his personal experience in volunteers and reported his findings to the medical community in 1958.[26] What does the presence of DMT in *Cohoba* have to do with ayahuasca? The answer came some years later when DMT was found in *Psychotria viridis*. But if DMT is inactive when taken by mouth, as Szara had shown, how do we account for the activity of ayahuasca tea? In the answer to that question lies the stroke of genius, some say the intervention of the gods, that led to the combination of *Psychotria viridis*, the source of DMT, and *Banisteriopsis caapi*. Contained in the latter plant is a family of chemicals called the *beta*-carbolines. Some members of the family are hallucinogenic, but their most significant contribution to ayahuasca is the fact that they inhibit an enzyme called monoamine oxidase (MAO). When taken by mouth, DMT is quickly inactivated by MAO. By blocking the enzyme, the carbolines permit DMT to reach the brain in adequate quantities. (Monoamine oxidase inhibitors were widely used in the 1950s for the treatment of depression. Whether an antidepressant action contributes to the overall effects of ayahuasca remains unknown.)

DMT, DR. STRASSMAN, AND MYSTICISM

No account of DMT would be complete without a discussion of the work of Rick Strassman. A psychiatrist by training, Strassman is the author of *DMT, The Spirit Molecule: A Doctor's Revolutionary Research Into the Biology of Near-Death and Mystical Experiences*.[27] The book, published in 2001, relates his observations of the effects of DMT in volunteers over a period of 5 years beginning in 1990. *DMT, The Spirit Molecule* brought the drug to the attention of the general public just as Aldous Huxley's *The Doors of Perception* had done for mescaline a half century earlier.

In November 1990, at the University of New Mexico Hospital Clinical Research Center, the first of Strassman's volunteers received an intravenous dose of DMT. This followed a 2-year struggle to surmount barriers imposed by various committees and bureaucrats of the University, the Food and Drug Administration, and the Drug Enforcement Administration; Strassman later described the process as Kafkaesque.[28] DMT was and is, we must recall, a Schedule I drug officially designated as having no medical use, lack of safety even under medical supervision, and a high probability of abuse. But, succeed he did, and, over the next 5 years, more than 400 doses of DMT were given to nearly five dozen men and women.

The first in a series of papers by Strassman appeared in 1994, a full 37 years after the initial report of the effects of DMT by Stephen Szara. Reminiscent of Szara's findings, Strassman's volunteers reported " . . . a rapidly moving, multi-dimensional, kaleidoscopic display of intensely colored abstract and representational images . . . "[29] What made these observations particularly provocative was the fact that, beginning in 1955, numerous studies had reported the presence of DMT and related chemicals in human blood, urine, and cerebrospinal fluid.[30] Based on these observations, it was hypothesized that DMT is an endogenous hallucinogen,[31] naturally produced in our brains and lungs, with a possible role in conditions such as schizophrenia; the latter suggestion was later dismissed by the psychiatric community on the basis that DMT did not fully mimic schizophrenia, that DMT was present in normal subjects, and assay methodology at that time could not differentiate between DMT levels in normal subjects and schizphrenics.[32]

Unfortunately, Strassman's research came to a virtual halt less than 6 years after his first volunteer had received DMT. He attributed this to a confluence of multiple negative factors. Among them were drug use by some of his staff, difficulty in recruiting others to join his team, and the constraints imposed by a strictly psychopharmacological model. These factors are familiar to any who have attempted to conduct human studies of a Schedule I hallucinogen such as DMT. Further complicating matters was Strassman's decision to accompany his former wife to Canada, where her family resided and where she was to receive cancer treatment. This necessitated supervision of the New Mexico studies from a distance, with Strassman spending only 2 weeks every 2 months in Albuquerque. The final blow came from an unexpected direction: his religious community.

Dr. Strassman had practiced and studied Zen Buddhism for decades and, in the 1990s maintained close contact with a California monastery. Indeed, he said that his understanding of Buddhism "pervaded nearly every aspect of working with The Spirit Molecule." However, an article he published in the Fall of 1996 in *Tricycle, The Buddhist Review*[33] met with condemnation by leaders of the monastic community. In it, Strassman had suggested that DMT might productively become a part of Buddhist practice and, reminiscent of Huxley's ideas about mescaline, might aid the dying. In a subsequent letter to Strassman, a leader of the monastery said that "Your psychedelic research is ultimately futile, devoid of real benefit to humanity, and dangerous . . . an attempt to induce enlightenment by chemical means can never, will never, succeed." Strassman's defeat was complete: ". . . the extra pressure exerted by my spiritual community broke down the last remnant of my desire to continue . . . I resigned from the University and returned the drugs to the National Institute on Drug Abuse . . ."[34]

This fraught ending does not diminish the contributions made by Strassman. His tenacity in overcoming the legal and bureaucratic barriers to the study of Schedule I drugs provided a model for all those who would follow. His studies of the dose–response relationship for DMT, demonstration of absence of tolerance to the drug, and preliminary mechanistic studies were the first of their kind. Fortunately for the science of psychedelics, Strassman later rekindled his investigative career, returned to the University of New Mexico School of Medicine, and has made further contributions to our understanding of DMT. These have included collaboration with a group seeking more sensitive assays for DMT and the development of an infusion protocol to permit a prolonged DMT experience.[35] A study assessing the functional status of members of an American branch of the *Uniao do Vegetal* who are regular users of DMT-containing ayahuasca found enhanced mood and reduced use of alcohol and marijuana.[36] In a preliminary but very provocative study of alcoholics, Strassman and his colleagues found that psilocybin treatment in combination with psychotherapy was followed by a significant increase in abstinence which was still present at 36-week follow-up.[37]

In *DMT, The Spirit Molecule*, Strassman tells us that he "was drawn to DMT because of its presence in all of our bodies." He then went on to speculate as to the source of DMT and its possible functions.

> The most general hypothesis is that the pineal gland produces psychedelic amounts of DMT at extraordinary times in our lives. . . . When our individual life force enters our fetal body, the moment in which we become truly human, it passes through the pineal and triggers the first primordial flood of DMT. . . . In some of us, pineal DMT mediates the pivotal experiences of deep meditation, psychosis, and near-death experiences. . . . As we die, the life-force leaves the body through the pineal gland, releasing another flood of this psychedelic spirit molecule.[38]

The pineal is a tiny organ situated deep in our brains, weighing just four thousandths of an ounce in adult humans. Rene Descartes called it the "seat of the soul" and Strassman points out that the "both Western and Eastern mystical traditions place our highest spiritual center within its confines." Modern physiology's view of the pineal is more pedestrian. It is well established that the gland is the source of melatonin, a hormone whose chemical structure resembles that of DMT. However, unlike DMT, melatonin has no hallucinogenic properties. Synthesis and release of melatonin are regulated by the light-dark cycle; light falling on the retina triggers signals which pass through a group of neurons called the suprachiasmatic nucleus and on to the pineal. Stimulated by darkness and inhibited by light, the waxing and waning of melatonin levels are correlated with our circadian rhythms, those regular fluctuations in sleepiness, body temperature, hormone release, and other bodily functions. In addition, melatonin has become a popular over-the-counter drug as a sleep aid and antidote for jet lag.

Earlier in this chapter, we met Aldous Huxley and his account of the mescaline experience in *The Doors of Perception*. It was Huxley's grandfather,

Thomas Henry Huxley, a 19th-century biologist noted for his defense of Darwin's theory of evolution, who spoke of "The great tragedy of science— the slaying of a beautiful hypothesis by an ugly fact." And that brings us back to Strassman's hypotheses on the role of the pineal and DMT. Writing in 2018, David Nichols, the pharmacologist and chemist who provided all of the synthetic DMT for Strassman's studies, concluded the following: "It is clear that very minute concentrations of DMT have been detected in the brain, but they are not sufficient to produce psychoactive effects."[39] To his credit, Strassman has expressed concern, both in *DMT, The Spirit Molecule* and in his subsequent writings, that too many assume "that the things I conjecture about are true."[40] They were instead intended to stimulate further research.

A BANKER AND THE *FLESH OF THE GODS*

We have already considered two classical hallucinogens that came to us from south of our border: mescaline of the peyote cactus and DMT in hallucinogenic snuffs. But our southern neighbors were to give us still another. When the Spaniards invaded Mexico in the 16th century, they found, among many other marvels, sculptured stones celebrating a kind of mushroom used in religious, sacrificial, and healing ceremonies. Archeologists would later establish that some of these monuments were more than 5,000 years old. In the Aztec Empire, the mushroom was called *teonanacatl*, the divine mushroom or, more colorfully, *flesh of the gods*. Not unlike their reaction to the use of peyote by the natives, the invading Spaniards regarded the mushroom cult as the work of Satan. Bernardino de Sahagun, whom we met earlier in his writings about peyote, said of teonanacatl that it "induced supernatural visions and even sexual ecstasy."[41] Not surprisingly, the Spanish conquerors banned the use of both peyote and teonanacatl in 1521.

Over the course of the next several centuries, science paid little attention to teonanacatl and, indeed, there was some confusion as to whether it and peyote were separate entities. It was not until early in the 20th century that the issue was settled when it was shown that the origin of teonanacatl was indeed a mushroom and thus quite distinct from mescaline and the peyote cactus.[42] The genus was given the name *Psilocybe* from the Greek for "bald or smooth head," an apt description both of the mushroom itself and the sculptures erected in its honor.

I have provided to you the names of many scientists and physicians over the course of the preceding pages, but it was a Wall Street banker, a member of the board of J.P. Morgan, who would bring teonanacatl to the attention of the world. R. Gordon Wasson and his new bride Valentina Pavlovna Guercken, born in Russia and a pediatrician by training, spent their honeymoon in the Catskill Mountains of New York State. There they encountered mushrooms reminiscent of those in Valentina's homeland. She loved them, he not so much. Nearly 30 years later, they learned of the divine mushroom of Mexico. Subsequently, they traveled to Mexico on numerous occasions, learned the Mazatec language, and ultimately they, together with their daughter, were permitted to take part in a teonanacatl ceremony. It took place on June 29, 1955. This is Gordon Wasson's description of the experience:

> We saw visions with our eyes open or closed, as if they sprang from a center point, sometimes faster, sometimes slower, in vibrant colors and artistic motifs in complete harmony, geometric figures and patterns as in rugs or carpets; then they changed into palaces adorned with gemstones with interior courtyards, colonnades, and gardens of supernatural splendor.[43]

An account of the teonanacatl experiences of Gordon Wasson was provided to the general public by *Life* magazine for May 13, 1957.[44] The title of the article was "Seeking the Magic Mushroom." But magic was not Gordon Wasson's line; in his writings he called the mushrooms divine, wondrous, sacred, and hallucinogenic but never magic. Nonetheless, *Life's* adjective stuck.

ALBERT HOFMANN AND THE SECRET OF THE MAGIC MUSHROOM

If some find magic in these fungi, what is its chemical origin? The year prior to the publication of "Seeking the Magic Mushroom," Gordon Wasson asked Roger Heim, director of the French National Museum of Natural History and a mycologist, an expert on mushrooms, to accompany him and Valentina to Mexico. During that trip, Heim identified several species of mushroom, including one given the name *Psilocybe mexicana Heim*. It was samples of that plant that Heim, in June 1957, personally delivered to Albert Hofmann in Basel.[45]

Tests of the effects of *Psilocybe mexicana* in mice and dogs were unimpressive. At that time, methods had not yet been developed to identify hallucinogens in animals.[46] Experiments in humans were needed. The estimable Dr. Hofmann would again serve as the human guinea pig. On July 1, 1957, he ate 2.4 grams of *Psilocybe mexicana.*

> After one half hour, the external world became unfamiliar. . . At the height of
> my intoxication, about one and one-half hours after ingesting the mushrooms,
> the onrushing images—mostly abstract motifs that rapidly shifted in form and
> color—became so intense that I feared being swept away and drawn into them and
> losing myself. Around six hours later, the dream ended. . . . Reentry into familiar
> reality was a welcome return home from a strange world that seemed so real.[47]

Hofmann and his colleagues at Sandoz then extracted a number of chemicals from the mushrooms and, using self-administration as a means to identify active components, soon had in hand the hallucinogenic essence of teonanacatl. Hofmann gave it the name *psilocybin.*[48] Eight months later he determined its chemical structure to be O-phosphoryl-4-hydroxy-*N,N*-dimethyltryptamine, a close relative of Szara's DMT.[49] Still simpler is psilocin, 4-hydroxy-DMT, the compound to which psilocybin is converted in our bodies. In the 1960s, Sandoz marketed psilocybin with the trade name Indocybin in tablets and capsules for use in conjunction with psychotherapy and psychoanalysis—a prelude to today's drug trials to be discussed later.

HALLUCINOGENS: DRUGS OF ABUSE
OR DRUG THERAPY

Our catalog of classical hallucinogens is now complete: mescaline, DMT, LSD, psilocybin. Comparison of the descriptions provided by Arthur Heffter, Stephen Szara, Albert Hofmann, and Gordon Wasson reveal that, despite some differences, the primarily visual distortions produced by the four drugs are quite similar as are their unique mental effects. As I noted earlier, we now believe that the four drugs share a common serotonergic mechanism of action.

How did these chemicals descend from being items of great scientific interest and, some believed, of great therapeutic potential, to being condemned as Schedule I drugs devoid of medical value and subject to a high probability of abuse? The answer to this question, as with so many others surrounding the drugs we love, is not to be found entirely in pharmacology. Social factors are at least as important. Some lay the blame at the feet of Timothy Leary.

TIMOTHY LEARY: THE PSILOCYBIN PROJECT

In 1960, Timothy Leary was a promising young psychologist who recently had been appointed to the faculty of Harvard University. As the author of a well-regarded book entitled *The Interpersonal Diagnosis of Personality*, the central question occupying Leary was how to change human behavior in a more efficient manner than was permitted by the psychotherapeutic methods then available. David McClelland, the director of the Center for Personality Research at Harvard, agreed to permit Leary to conduct a project to examine the question; the details of the project were yet to be developed. That same year, while on vacation in Mexico, Leary had his first experience with a hallucinogenic drug. It was psilocybin contained in Wasson's magic mushrooms.

> The journey lasted a little over four hours. Like almost everyone who has had the veil drawn, I came back a changed man. . . . In four hours . . . I learned more about the mind, the brain, and its structures than I did in the preceding fifteen years as a diligent psychologist . . . a deeply religious experience.[50]

Thus was born what was to be called the Harvard Psilocybin Project. Rather than mushrooms, pure psilocybin, provided by Sandoz, was to be used. The initial experiments involved 38 persons recruited largely from among Harvard graduate students and faculty; the number would later grow to more than 200. Nearly all found the sessions, many of which were conducted in Leary's home, to be pleasant and "consciousness expanding." Leary believed that he had discovered a route to "instant psychoanalysis." The following year, firm in his belief that long-term behavioral changes could be induced by psilocybin, Leary began what was to be called the Concord Prison Psilocybin Rehabilitation Project. Convicts in this Massachusetts prison were treated with psilocybin in group therapy sessions followed by extensive psychological testing. The crucial end point was the rate of recidivism. Leary reported that the rate fell from the historical average of 70% to less than 25%.[51] (A later analysis of Leary's data contested this conclusion.[52])

LSD: THE ACADEMIC RISE AND FALL OF DR. LEARY

Today, Timothy Leary's name is most often associated, not with psilocybin, but with LSD. Initially, Leary was wary of LSD as a synthetic chemical, believing it inferior to psilocybin with its natural source in mushrooms and its long history in American Indian culture. His attitude changed dramatically in 1962 when Leary experienced the effects of LSD for the first time.

> Psilocybin had let me spiral down the DNA ladder of evolution up to the beginning of life on the planet. But LSD was something different . . . (it) had flipped my consciousness into a dance of energy, where nothing existed except whirring vibrations . . . it was the most shattering experience of my life.[53]

From that time on, LSD was Leary's drug of choice.

Meanwhile, back on the Harvard campus, things were getting a bit more complicated. Students began taking psilocybin and LSD outside the bounds of defined experiments; many, it was suggested, with the complicity of Dr. Leary. It did not help that LSD was increasingly associated with sexual activity, always a parental concern. Recall that 400 years earlier Bernardino de Sahagun wrote that teonanacatl "induced supernatural visions and even sexual ecstasy." Leary would later call LSD "the most powerful aphrodisiac ever discovered by man." The Harvard administration, initially pleased with the results of the psilocybin projects, became increasingly uneasy about the publicity surrounding Leary's activities. On May 6, 1963, Harvard's president terminated Leary's university appointment.

LSD ENTERS THE MAINSTREAM

Despite the very great influence exerted by Timothy Leary prior to and following his dismissal from Harvard, I believe that the real driver of the rise of LSD was a matter of supply. Although Sandoz had denied Leary's request to purchase 100 grams of LSD and 55 pounds of psilocybin, American chemists took up the gauntlet. First among these were Melissa Cargill and her partner, Owsley Stanley, a self-taught chemist. Together they synthesized several million doses of the drug and were the suppliers of LSD to, among many others, The Grateful Dead. Still more productive was Nicholas Sand, a protégé of Tim Scully, laboratory partner of Stanley. Near the end of his life, Sand claimed to have produced in Canada and the United States some 140 million doses of LSD.

With increasing availability of LSD came increasing governmental scrutiny. In 1962, the Food and Drug Administration designated LSD as an experimental drug and imposed restrictions on research. Four years later, outright illegality of LSD was declared by the State of California to be followed by a national ban in 1968. Public Law 90-639 amended the Food, Drug, and Cosmetic Act to explicitly include LSD. Mere possession of the drug could be punished by up to 1 year in prison; sale of LSD could draw a 10-year sentence. It was under these provisions that Owsley Stanley, Tim Scully, and Nicholas Sand would later spend significant time in federal prison. Finally, the Comprehensive Drug Abuse Prevention and Control Act of 1970 created a scheduling system for drugs. Mescaline, DMT, and psilocybin, along with LSD, were placed in Schedule I as having no accepted medical use and a high potential for abuse.

HALLUCINOGENS AND THERAPY

Despite the long shadow cast by our legal system in placing the hallucinogens in Schedule I, Albert Hofmann's dream that LSD and psilocybin would find a place in medicine has endured. Indeed, there is today hope on the part of some that it will be fulfilled. This hope comes not so much from new hypotheses but instead from the rigorous testing of what, for the most part, are old ideas. At the heart of these ideas is the thought, expressed more than a century ago by Silas Weir Mitchell following his experience with peyote, that drugs such as this could "release a mob of verbal memories."[54] Put another way, repressed memories might be brought to the surface and dealt with by traditional psychotherapy (The less formal term is "talk therapy.") Current studies of hallucinogens in treating obsessive-compulsive disorders, posttraumatic stress disorder, and a variety of addictions seek to exploit this effect.

In describing Timothy Leary's experiences at Harvard, I may have given the impression that his thoughts on LSD were original with him. They were not. In the 15 years between Werner Stoll's account of the effects of LSD in normal persons and psychiatric patients and Leary's first experience with LSD in 1962, more than a thousand publications on LSD appeared in the scientific literature. Although of uneven quality, these studies, taken together, permitted several broad conclusions to be drawn regarding LSD: (1) latent psychosis may be triggered and pre-existing psychosis may be worsened, (2) coupled with psychotherapy, anxiety and depression may be lifted, and (3) beneficial effects appear to linger long after the drug has left the body. More controversial were suggestions that sexual deviancy, which at that time included homosexuality, could be cured. Also emerging was the view that use of LSD in a nonmedical setting could be dangerous, especially in someone unfamiliar with its effects. We are reminded of Hofmann's comment following his first intentional exposure to LSD: "A terrible fear that I had lost my mind grabbed me."[55] It is true that, in contrast with the virtually nonexistent direct toxic effects of LSD, irrational behavior while intoxicated sometimes has had lethal consequences. It is for this reason that, in today's therapeutic trials of hallucinogens, emphasis is placed on the mental and physical state of the subject, the set, and the environment in which the drug is given, the setting.

Six days after the appearance in 1955 of *Life* magazine's "The Magic Mushroom," a similar article appeared in *This Week*, a supplement to numerous Sunday papers. In it, Valentina Pavlovna Wasson suggested a range of possible uses for psilocybin-containing mushrooms. A particularly intriguing thought was that the mushrooms might provide comfort to the dying. With Hofmann's identification of psilocybin that same year, it became possible to test Wasson's idea with a pure hallucinogen. A prominent advocate of such studies was Aldous Huxley, who wrote that "the living can do a great deal to make the passage easier for the dying." Several hours before his own death in 1963 from cancer, Huxley asked for LSD. His wife, Laura, injected 100 micrograms of the drug. He is said to have died peacefully a few hours later. In contrast, Albert Hofmann declined the use of the drug at the time of his death on April 29, 2008, at the age of 102. A week before, he had said that "I don't think I need LSD to die; I can face death with joy. I am looking forward to seeing my relatives and friends again."[56]

Studies conducted in the 1950s and 1960s of hallucinogens as comfort for the dying were quite different from Huxley's experience in that LSD or psilocybin was given on multiple occasions and always accompanied by psychotherapy. The results were encouraging but, with the placing of hallucinogens in Schedule I, such investigations soon ended. It was still possible to get permission to study the drugs in humans, but the bureaucratic hurdles to be cleared remained formidable. Furthermore, federal granting agencies had little interest in providing financial support; investigators were better advised to seek adverse effects of the hallucinogens. Nonetheless, some continued to carry the torch and, in recent years, well-designed studies to measure relief of anxiety and depression in patients suffering life-threatening cancer have yielded positive results.[575859] The prospect of wider application in the general population remains uncertain.

THE GOOD FRIDAY EXPERIMENT AND ITS SUCCESSORS

The final issue we shall address with respect to hallucinogens is nicely introduced by Aldous Huxley in *The Doors of Perception*.

> The man who comes back through the Door in the Wall will never be quite the same as the man who went out. He will be wiser but less sure, happier but less

self-satisfied, humbler in acknowledging his ignorance yet better equipped to understand the relationship of words to things, of systematic reasoning to the unfathomable mystery which it tries, forever vainly, to comprehend.[60]

Might these drugs in fact be psychedelic as Osmond defined the word: enriching the mind and enlarging the vision? Might they induce mystical experiences? Might their effects, as Huxley suggests, persist long after the drugs have left the body? These are not contentions easily proven. One who tried was Walter Pahnke.

Already a graduate of Harvard University's schools of medicine and divinity, Pahnke was, in 1962, a PhD candidate at Harvard. His mentor was Timothy Leary. That year, 2 days before Easter Sunday, they conducted what came to be called the Good Friday Experiment in the Marsh Chapel of Boston University. Their subjects were 20 white male Christian divinity students at the Andover Newton Theological School who had no previous experience with psilocybin or other psychoactive drugs. Split into two groups, 10 received capsules containing psilocybin, and the others nicotinic acid to serve as a control. The students then attended a 2-hour religious service. Psilocybin had been chosen for use rather than LSD because of the former's shorter duration of action. To assess the effects of the drug, Pahnke devised what he called "a mystical experience questionnaire" designed to test "seven domains of mystical experiences." Subjects completed the questionnaire shortly after the psilocybin experiment and again 6 months later.

In June 1963, Pahnke presented the results of the Good Friday Experiment to his Harvard PhD committee in a thesis titled *Drugs and Mysticism: An Analysis of the Relationship Between Psychedelic Drugs and the Mystical Consciousness*.[61] In it, he described how nine of the ten students who received psilocybin had "deeply moving and religious experiences." Six months later, eight of the ten students reported that positive effects of the drug persisted in their daily lives.[62,63] Still more remarkable, a meticulous follow-up study conducted a quarter century later found "a substantial amount of persisting positive effects and no significant long-term negative effects."[64]

More than a half century has passed since completion of the Good Friday Experiment. During that period, a number of studies were conducted in attempts to establish a relationship between hallucinogenic drugs and mystical experiences. Most prominent among them are those conducted by Roland Griffiths, professor of psychiatry and behavioral sciences in the Johns Hopkins University School of Medicine. Griffiths has long been a world leader in the study of drug-induced mysticism.

In August 2006, an article was published by Griffiths and his colleagues in *Psychopharmacology*, a well-regarded international journal devoted, as its name implies, to the study of psychoactive drugs both in animals and in humans. The title of the article was "Psilocybin Can Occasion Mystical-Type Experiences Having Substantial and Sustained Personal Meaning and Spiritual Significance."[65] It was an appropriate place to report Griffiths's findings; the initial issue of the journal 47 years earlier (it was then called *Psychopharmacologia*) contained an article from investigators at the United States Narcotic Farm in Lexington, Kentucky, discussed in chapter 2, on the effects of psilocybin and LSD in their prisoner "volunteers." Despite *Psychopharmcologia*'s long history with such drugs, the mention of mysticism and spirituality led to an unusual move by the journal editors in soliciting commentary from four leading authorities on hallucinogens.

Thirty-six volunteers recruited from the Baltimore area received psilocybin and methylphenidate in sessions 2 months apart. From chapter 4, you will recall that methylphenidate (Ritalin) is an amphetamine-like stimulant widely used to treat attention-deficit/hyperactivity disorder. Thirty of the subjects were divided into two groups of 15 each. One group received psilocybin in the first session followed by methylphenidate in the second. The order was reversed for the other 15. Six additional subjects received methylphenidate in the first two sessions and psilocybin in a third session. All experiments were done in a "living-room-like" setting in the presence of two experienced monitors who, like the volunteers, were not told what drug had been given; that is, the design was "double-blind." Eye masks and classical music via headphones were available if desired. None of the subjects had had previous experience with hallucinogenic drugs, nearly all had completed college, more than half had postgraduate degrees, and all had previously participated in religious or spiritual activities.

Seven hours after drug administration, the subjects completed multiple questionnaires to assess hallucinogenic effects and "altered states of consciousness." The latter included a scale measuring "oceanic boundlessness, a state common to classical mystical experiences including feelings of unity and transcendence of time and space." Two months after drug treatments, the subjects were again evaluated, via questionnaires, about any persisting effects of the drugs.

Twenty-two of the 36 subjects had, by the criteria of the investigators, "complete mystical experiences" induced by psilocybin, while only four of the 36 did so following methylphenidate. More than three quarters rated the psilocybin experience as either the most significant or among the top-five most significant "spiritual experiences of their lives." An independent assessment was provided by what were called "community observers." Each volunteer had designated three family members, friends, or coworkers who were asked to comment on what they perceived as changes in the subjects' behavior, attitudes, and values. Immediately after psilocybin administration, positive effects were reported by both the volunteers and the community observers. Quite remarkably, these were maintained, in somewhat diminished force, 2 months after psilocybin administration and were still detectable after 14 months.[66] In a subsequent study, psilocybin administration was coupled with a guided program of meditation and other spiritual practices.[67] The results were as before, and the positive effects were still present at 6-month follow-up.

The professionals asked to comment on the 2006 investigation were united in praising the rigor of the study. They noted the exclusion of volunteers with prior experience with hallucinogens, the counseling of the subjects prior to drug administration, the provision of guides during the experience, the use of a double-blind design, the inclusion of methylphenidate as a positive control, and extensive follow-up over many months.

David Nichols, the pharmacologist and chemist who had synthesized the psilocybin used in the study, saw the investigation as a significant extension of and improvement upon the Pahnke Good Friday Experiment. Solomon Snyder, professor of neuroscience at the Johns Hopkins University School of Medicine, observed that psychoactive plant extracts have been in use for religious purposes for thousands of years and continue to this day in groups such as the Native American Church and Uniao de Vegetal. He expressed the view that reliable production of a mystical state might lead to an understanding of the molecular alterations in the brain that underlie religious experiences. The Griffiths group had commented that the psilocybin-induced state was similar to spontaneously occurring mystical experiences. No longer dependent on achieving the mystical state by traditional approaches such as prolonged fasting, chanting, solitude, or meditation, the drug would permit rigorous scientific investigations of the phenomenon.

Herbert Kleber, professor of psychiatry at Columbia University's College of Physicians and Surgeons and author of a textbook on addiction treatment, spoke of the profound therapeutic role in the treatment of addictive disorders of spiritual awakening, whether arising from religion, 12-step programs such as that of Alcoholic Anonymous, or a profound life experience.

On a cautionary note, Dr. Kleber also suggested that reports of positive effects might lead to increased use of drugs like psilocybin by inexperienced enlightenment seekers, especially the young, in uncontrolled settings. In that respect, I suspect that the horse is already out of the barn as we find best-selling authors such as Michael Pollan describing his self-experiments with LSD, psilocybin mushrooms, and the DMT of ayahuasca in generally glowing terms; I say "generally glowing" because Pollan also notes periods of anxiety and even terror.[68] Maria Estavez, a participant in Griffiths's studies, wrote an article about her psilocybin experience in which she said that "it was if a light was revealing to me the innermost workings of the universe."[69]

Adventurous readers inclined to replicate Mr. Pollan's self-experiments should be reminded of the continued illegality of the hallucinogens. While it is true that police in recent years have often looked the other way regarding enforcement of the law, the potential penalties for users remain harsh. For example, use of LSD remains punishable by imprisonment under both state and federal law. The federal penalty is a maximum of 1 year in prison and a fine of $1,000. State laws are even more draconian; mere possession in Louisiana is punishable by up to 10 years of hard labor.

IF THE HUMAN BRAIN WERE SO SIMPLE

As I have noted earlier and as I will repeat in the chapter that follows, the evidence supporting a potential value of hallucinogens, particularly psilocybin, as an adjunct to psychotherapy is compelling. Practical applications, for which substantial supporting evidence already exists, include the treatment of anxiety and depression, especially that associated with the end of life, posttraumatic stress disorder, and for a variety of addictive states, including nicotine, alcohol, and opioid dependence. But it must be emphasized that all such applications are in conjunction with psychotherapy, a therapeutic modality which continues to be a prolonged and labor-intensive process; there is no evidence that the hallucinogens can stand alone. As to revealing "the innermost workings of the universe," I remain agnostic. Furthermore, I believe that our brains are sufficiently complex to support all sorts of quasi-mystical drug-induced experiences without the need to invoke supernatural forces. Will we at some time in the future have a complete understanding of the secrets of our nervous systems? Perhaps, but I am reminded of a thought expressed many years ago by Emerson M. Pugh and quoted by his son George: If the human brain were so simple that we could understand it, we would be so simple that we couldn't.[70]

NOTES

1. Schultes RE, Hofmann A (1980) *The Botany and Chemistry of Hallucinogens.* Springfield, IL: Charles C. Thomas.
2. Lewin L (1924) *Phantastika-die Betaubenden und erregenden Genussmittle.* Berlin: Verlag G. Stilke. Lewin L (1964) *Phantastica-Narcotic and Stimulating Drugs—Their Use and Abuse.* London: Routledge & Kegan Paul.
3. Osmond H (1957) A review of the clinical effects of psychotomimetic agents. *Ann NY Acad Sci* 66(3):418–434.
4. Fiorella D, Rabin RA, Winter JC 1995) The role of the 5-HT$_{2A}$ and 5-HT$_{2C}$ receptors in the stimulus effects of hallucinogenic drugs I: Antagonist correlation analysis. *Psychopharmacology* 121:347–356.
5. Nichols DE (2016) Psychedelics. *Pharmacol Rev* 68:264–355.
6. Schultes RE, Hofmann A (1980) *The Botany and Chemistry of Hallucinogens.* Springfield, IL: Charles C. Thomas.
7. Sahagan B (1938) Vol 3 of *Historia general de las Cosas de la Nueva Espana.* Editorial Pedro Robledo. Mexico, D.F.
8. Mitchell SW (1896) Remarks on the effects of Anhelonium Lewinii (The Mescal Button). *Brit Med J* Dec. 5:1625–1628.
9. Ellis H (1897) A note on the phenomena of mescal intoxication. *The Lancet* I(3849):1540–1542.
10. Ellis H (1898) Mescal: A new artificial paradise. *The Contemporary Review* 74:130–141.
11. Heffter A (1897) Ueber Pellote. *Arch Exp Path Pharmacol* 40:418–425. English translation in Holmstedt B, Liljestrand (1963) *Readings in Pharmacology.* London: Pergamon Press.
12. Huxley A (1954) *The Doors of Perception.* New York: Harper & Brothers.
13. Hacker MS (2018) Parker, Cynthia Parker. *Handbook of Texas Online.* Accessed June 29, 2018. http://www.tshaonline.org/handbook/online/articles/fpa18.
14. Hagenbach D, Werthmuller L (2013) *Mystical Chemist: The Life of Albert Hofmann and His Discovery of LSD.* Santa Fe, NM: Synergetic Press. Throughout this section on Hofmann and his discoveries regarding LSD and psilocybin, I have drawn extensively from *Mystical Chemist,* a book which, in my experience, is unsurpassed in providing details of the personal life and career of this remarkable man. More limited but having the virtue of being Hofmann's personal account is *LSD, My Problem Child: Reflections on Sacred Drugs, Mysticism and Science.* Originally published in German as *LSD: Mein Sorgenkind,* the book was republished in an English edition with additional materials in 2009 by the Multidisciplinary Association for Psychedelic Studies.
15. Anonymous (1955) The history of LSD 25 (lysergic acid diethylamide). *Sandoz J Med Sci* II(3):117–124.
16. Anonymous (1955) The history of LSD 25 (lysergic acid diethylamide). *Sandoz J Med Sci* II(3):117–124.
17. Anonymous (1955) The history of LSD 25 (lysergic acid diethylamide). *Sandoz J Med Sci* II(3):117–124.
18. Anonymous (1955) The history of LSD 25 (lysergic acid diethylamide). *Sandoz J Med Sci* II(3):117–124.
19. Anonymous (1955) The history of LSD 25 (lysergic acid diethylamide). *Sandoz J Med Sci* II(3):117–124.

20. Hagenbach D, Werthmuller L (2013) *Mystical Chemist: The Life of Albert Hofmann and His Discovery of LSD*. Santa Fe, NM: Synergetic Press. Throughout this section on Hofmann and his discoveries regarding LSD and psilocybin, I have drawn extensively from *Mystical Chemist*, a book which, in my experience, is unsurpassed in providing details of the personal life and career of this remarkable man. More limited but having the virtue of being Hofmann's personal account is *LSD, My Problem Child: Reflections on Sacred Drugs, Mysticism and Science*. Originally published in German as *LSD: Mein Sorgenkind*, the book was republished in an English edition with additional materials in 2009 by the Multidisciplinary Association for Psychedelic Studies.

21. Stoll W (1947) *Lysergsäure-diathylämid, ein Phantastikum aus der Mutterkorngruppe"* (Lysergic acid diethylamide, a phantasticum from the ergot group). *Schweizer Archiv fur Neurologie und Psychiatrie (Swiss Archives of Neurology and Psychiatry)* 60:279–286.

22. Schultes RE, Hofmann A (1980) *The Botany and Chemistry of Hallucinogens*. Springfield, IL: Charles C. Thomas.

23. Gill V (2006) Jungle fever: An ayahuasca healing retreat. *The Sunday Times*, January 8.

24. Szara S (2007) DMT at fifty. *Neuropsychopharmacol Hung* 9(4):201–205.

25. Fish MS, Johnson NM, Horning EC (1955) *Piptadenia* alkaloids. Indole bases of *P. peregrine* (L.) Benth and related species. *J Am Chem Soc* 77:5892–5895.

26. Sai-Halasz A Von, Brunecker G, Szara S (1958) Dimethyltripamin: Ein neus Psychoticum. *Psychiat Neurol Basel* 135:285–301.

27. Strassman, RJ (2001) *DMT, The Spirit Molecule: A Doctor's Revolutionary Research Into the Biology of Near-Death and Mystical Experiences*. Rochester, VT: Park Street Press.

28. Strassman, RJ (1991) Human hallucinogenic drug research in the United States: A present-day case history and review of the process. *J Psychoactive Drugs* 23 (1):29–38.

29. Strassman, RJ (1996) Human psychopharmacology of N,N-dimethyltryptamine. *Behav Brain Res* 73:121–124.

30. Barker, SA, McIllhenny, EH, Strassman, RJ (2012) A critical review of reports of endogenous psychedelic N,N-dimethyltryptamines in humans: 1955–2010. *Drug Test Analysis* 4:617–635.

31. Barker, SA, Monti, JA, Christian, ST (1981) N-N-Dimethyltryptamine: An endogenous hallucinogen. *Int Rev Neurobiol* 22:83–110.

32. Gillin, JC, Kaplan J, Stillman R, Wyatt, RJ (1976) The psychedelic model of schizophrenia: The case of N,N-Dimethyltryptamine. *Amer J Psychiatr* 133:203–208.

33. Strassman, RJ (1996) DMT and the Dharma. *Tricycle, The Buddhist Review* 6:81–88.

34. Strassman, RJ (2001) *DMT, The Spirit Molecule: A Doctor's Revolutionary Research Into the Biology of Near-Death and Mystical Experiences*. Rochester, VT: Park Street Press.

35. Gallimore AR, Strassman RJ (2016) A model for the application of target-controlled intravenous infusion for a prolonged immersive DMT psychedelic experience. *Front Pharmacol* 7:211–216.

36. Barbosa PC, Strassman RJ, da Silveira DX, Areco K, Hoy R, Pommy J, Thoma R, Bogenschutz M. (2016). Psychological and neuropsychological assessment of regular hoasca users. *Compr Psychiatry* 21:95–105.

37. Bogenschutz MP, Forcehimes AA, Pommy JA, Wilcox CE, Barbosa PC, Strassman RJ (2015) Psilocybin-assisted treatment for alcohol dependence: A proof-of-concept study. *J Psychopharmacol* 29(3):289–299.

38. Strassman, RJ (2001) *DMT, The Spirit Molecule: A Doctor's Revolutionary Research Into the Biology of Near-Death and Mystical Experiences.* Rochester, VT: Park Street Press.

39. Nichols, DE (2018) N,N-Dimethyltryptamine and the pineal gland: Separating fact from myth. *J Psychopharmacol* 32 (1):30–36.

40. Hanna, J (2017) DMT and the pineal: Fact of fiction. Erowid.org/chemicals/dmt/dmt_article2.stml

41. Sahagan B (1938) Vol 3 of *Historia general de las Cosas de la Nueva Espana.* Editorial Pedro Robledo. Mexico, D.F.

42. Schultes RE, Hofmann A (1980) *The Botany and Chemistry of Hallucinogens.* Springfield, IL: Charles C. Thomas.

43. Wasson VP, Wasson RG (1957) *Mushrooms, Russia and History.* New York: Pantheon Books.

44. Wasson RG (1957) Seeking the Magic Mushroom. *Life,* May 13. www.imaginaria.org/wasson/life.htm

45. Hagenbach D, Werthmuller L (2013) *Mystical Chemist: The Life of Albert Hofmann and His Discovery of LSD.* Santa Fe, NM: Synergetic Press. Throughout this section on Hofmann and his discoveries regarding LSD and psilocybin, I have drawn extensively from *Mystical Chemist,* a book which, in my experience, is unsurpassed in providing details of the personal life and career of this remarkable man. More limited but having the virtue of being Hofmann's personal account is *LSD, My Problem Child: Reflections on Sacred Drugs, Mysticism and Science.* Originally published in German as *LSD: Mein Sorgenkind,* the book was republished in an English edition with additional materials in 2009 by the Multidisciplinary Association for Psychedelic Studies.

46. Winter JC (1971) Hallucinogens as discriminative stimuli. *Fed Proc* 33:1825–1832.

47. Hagenbach D, Werthmuller L (2013) *Mystical Chemist: The Life of Albert Hofmann and His Discovery of LSD.* Santa Fe, NM: Synergetic Press. Throughout this section on Hofmann and his discoveries regarding LSD and psilocybin, I have drawn extensively from *Mystical Chemist,* a book which, in my experience, is unsurpassed in providing details of the personal life and career of this remarkable man. More limited but having the virtue of being Hofmann's personal account is *LSD, My Problem Child: Reflections on Sacred Drugs, Mysticism and Science.* Originally published in German as *LSD: Mein Sorgenkind,* the book was republished in an English edition with additional materials in 2009 by the Multidisciplinary Association for Psychedelic Studies.

48. Hofmann A, Heim R, Brack A et al. (1958) Psilocybin, a psychotropic substance from the Mexican mushroom Psilocybe mexicana Heim. *Experientia* 14:107–109.

49. Hofmann A, Frey A, Ott H et al (1958) Elucidation of the structure and the synthesis of psilocybin. *Experientia* 14:397–399.

50. Leary T (1983) *Flashbacks: An Autobiography.* Boston: J.P. Tarcher.

51. Leary TF, Metzner R, Presnell M, Weil G, Schwitzgebel R, Kinne S (1965) A new behavior change program for adult offenders using psilocybin. *Psychotherapy* 2(2):61–72.

52. Doblin R (1998) Dr. Leary's Concord Prison Experiment: A 34-year follow-up study. *J Psychoactive Drugs* 30(4):419–426.

53. Hagenbach D, Werthmuller L (2013) *Mystical Chemist: The Life of Albert Hofmann and His Discovery of LSD*. Santa Fe, NM: Synergetic Press. Throughout this section on Hofmann and his discoveries regarding LSD and psilocybin, I have drawn extensively from *Mystical Chemist*, a book which, in my experience, is unsurpassed in providing details of the personal life and career of this remarkable man. More limited but having the virtue of being Hofmann's personal account is *LSD, My Problem Child: Reflections on Sacred Drugs, Mysticism and Science*. Originally published in German as *LSD: Mein Sorgenkind*, the book was republished in an English edition with additional materials in 2009 by the Multidisciplinary Association for Psychedelic Studies.

54. Mitchell SW (1896) Remarks on the effects of Anhelonium Lewinii (The Mescal Button). *Brit Med J* Dec. 5:1625–1628.

55. Hagenbach D, Werthmuller L (2013) *Mystical Chemist: The Life of Albert Hofmann and His Discovery of LSD*. Santa Fe, NM: Synergetic Press. Throughout this section on Hofmann and his discoveries regarding LSD and psilocybin, I have drawn extensively from *Mystical Chemist*, a book which, in my experience, is unsurpassed in providing details of the personal life and career of this remarkable man. More limited but having the virtue of being Hofmann's personal account is *LSD, My Problem Child: Reflections on Sacred Drugs, Mysticism and Science*. Originally published in German as *LSD: Mein Sorgenkind*, the book was republished in an English edition with additional materials in 2009 by the Multidisciplinary Association for Psychedelic Studies.

56. Hagenbach D, Werthmuller L (2013) *Mystical Chemist: The Life of Albert Hofmann and His Discovery of LSD*. Santa Fe, NM: Synergetic Press. Throughout this section on Hofmann and his discoveries regarding LSD and psilocybin, I have drawn extensively from *Mystical Chemist*, a book which, in my experience, is unsurpassed in providing details of the personal life and career of this remarkable man. More limited but having the virtue of being Hofmann's personal account is *LSD, My Problem Child: Reflections on Sacred Drugs, Mysticism and Science*. Originally published in German as *LSD: Mein Sorgenkind*, the book was republished in an English edition with additional materials in 2009 by the Multidisciplinary Association for Psychedelic Studies.

57. Ross, S, Bossis A, Guss J, Agin-Liebes G, Malone T, Cohen B, Mennenga SE, Belser A, Kalliontzi K, Babb J, Su Z, Corby P, Schmidt BL (2016) Rapid and sustained symptom reduction following psilocybin treatment for anxiety and depression in patients with life-threatening cancer: A randomized controlled trial. *J Psychopharmacol* 30(12):1165–1180.

58. Spiegel D (2016) Psilocybin-assisted psychotherapy for dying cancer patients: Aiding the final trip. *J Pschopharmacol* 30(12):1215–1217.

59. Griffiths RR, Johnson MW, Carducci MA et al. (2016) Psilocybin produces substantial and sustained decreases in depression and anxiety in patients with life-threatening cancer: A randomized double-blind trial. *J Psychopharmacol* 30:1181–1197.

60. Huxley A (1954) *The Doors of Perception*. New York: Harper & Brothers.

61. Pahnke WN (1963) *Drugs and Mysticism: An Analysis of the Relationship Between Psychedelic Drugs and the Mystical Consciousness*. Cambridge, MA: Harvard University Press.

62. Pahnke WN, Richards WA (1966) Implications of LSD and experimental mysticism. *J Relig Health* 5(3):175–208.

63. Pahnke WN (1969) Psychedelic drugs and mystical experience. *Int Psychiatry Clin* 5(4):149–162.

64. Doblin R (1991) Pahnke's "Good Friday Experiment": A long-term follow-up and methodological critique. *J Transpersonal Psychol* 23(1):1–28.

65. Griffiths RR, Richards WA, McCann U, Jesse R (2006) Psilocybin can occasion mystical-type experiences having substantial and sustained personal meaning and spiritual significance. *Psychopharmacology* 187:268–283.

66. Griffiths R, Richards W, Johnson M, McCann U, Jesse R (2008) Mystical-type experiences occasioned by psilocybin mediate the attribution of personal meaning and spiritual significance 14 months later. *J Psychopharmacol* 22(6):621–632.

67. Griffifths RR, Johnson MW, Richards WA, Richards BD, Jesse R, MacLean KA, Barrett FS, Cosimano MP, Klinedinst MA (2018) Psilocybin-occasioned mystical-type experiences in combination with meditation and other spiritual practices produces enduring positive changes in psychological functioning and in trait measures of prosocial attitudes and behaviors. *J Psychopharmacol* 32(1):49–69.

68. Pollan M (2018) *How to Change Your Mind*. New York: Penguin Press.

69. Estavez M (2010) High light: When a psilocybin study leads to spiritual realization. *Sci Am* November 23, 2010.

70. Pugh GE (1977) *The Biological Origins of Human Values*. New York: Basic Books.

CHAPTER 8

cVo

Methylenedioxymethamphetamine (MDMA)

a.k.a. Ecstasy

As these words are written, the chemical we will call MDMA is a Schedule I drug. This means that MDMA (a) has no currently accepted medical use, (b) no currently accepted safety even under medical supervision, and (c) has a high potential for abuse. On the other hand, there are those who see great therapeutic potential in MDMA, and the Food and Drug Administration (FDA) has designated MDMA-assisted psychotherapy as a breakthrough therapy. We can foresee the day when it will be available by prescription.

There is no doubt as to the chemical identity of MDMA, and much is known of its pharmacological effects in humans and in animals. The recreational drug commonly known as Ecstasy is more complicated. As is true for any illegal drug used by millions of people, demand for the drug has been met by persons not noted for their high ethical or manufacturing standards. Simply stated, short of chemical analysis, one can never be sure what street-bought Ecstasy is. For example, investigators at Vanderbilt University determined the contents of 1,214 tablets sold as Ecstasy. Only 39% contained only MDMA, while fully 46% were "substances other than MDMA."[1] Mixtures of MDMA and other drugs comprised the remaining 15%. On the other hand, sometimes in some places over the past several decades, nearly pure MDMA has been available on the illicit market.

Our Love Affair with Drugs: The History, the Science, the Politics. Jerrold Winter, Oxford University Press (2020). © Jerrold Winter.
DOI: 10.1093/oso/9780190051464.001.0001

Nonetheless, a buyer of Ecstasy may ingest, rather than MDMA, drugs such as ketamine, *gamma*-hydroxybutyrate (GHB), cathinone, ephedrine, caffeine, or any one of the so-called designer drugs, many of which are amphetamine derivatives. A consequence of this pharmacological chaos is that many of the hazards associated with the use of Ecstasy have been uncritically attributed to MDMA. This fact has been a boon for those who would continue the Schedule I status of MDMA and a bane for those who would explore its therapeutic potential. However, in contrast with recreational use where purity of the drug is uncertain, MDMA in clinical trials is FDA approved and of known composition.

ALEXANDER SHULGUN: THE MAN WHO LOVED DRUGS

Before addressing these issues in detail, let us consider the history of MDMA and an extraordinary man named Alexander Shulgin. I first met the late Dr. Shulgin in 1998 at a meeting on psychedelics sponsored by the National Institute on Drug Abuse (NIDA). I was prepared to be intimidated. After all, he was by that time the author of many research papers and of two iconic books with the odd names of *PiHKAL* and *TiHKAL*. The first letters in the titles refer to phenethylamines and tryptamines. Representative members of the phenethylamine and tryptamine families are the hallucinogens, mescaline and DMT, respectively, which we met in chapter 7. *iHKAL* in both titles is the acronym for "I Have Known and Loved." In the books' nearly 1,800 pages we find descriptions, recipes if you will, for the synthesis of countless psychoactive drugs, including MDMA.[2,3] Still more remarkable is that Shulgin and his wife, Ann, provide accounts of their and their friends' personal experiences with these drugs. Although Alexander Shulgin had been called a chemical magician by some and a menace to society by others, intimidating he was not. Upon addressing him as Dr. Shulgin, he immediately told me to call him Sasha.

It is an understatement to say that Shulgin's methods were unconventional. You may recall that in chapter 3 we considered double-blind trials in which neither investigator nor subject is aware of drug and placebo assignments until after data are gathered. Such trials continue to be the gold standard for establishing proof of either benefit or risk of a given drug. In contrast, Shulgin once called his method "triple consciousness." He made the drug, he took the drug, and he would tell you what its effects were. MDMA was one of those drugs.

A native of California and a precocious student, Alexander Shulgin began his studies at Harvard College in 1941 at the age of 16 but soon dropped out to enlist in the Navy. After the war, he completed an under-graduate degree in organic chemistry and a PhD degree in biochemistry both at the University of California at Berkeley. As a research scientist at Dow Chemical, he developed a very successful line of pesticides. However, in 1960, Shulgin had experienced for the first time the effects of mesca-line, and his interests soon shifted to psychoactive drugs. Indeed, he syn-thesized MDMA while at Dow in 1965 but did not explore its effects at that time. Nine years would pass before MDMA would again come to his attention.

By 1976, having left Dow, Shulgin and his wife, Ann, had become, in the words of Rick Doblin, about whom we shall learn more in a mo-ment, "the core around which the California psychedelic community cohered."[4]

In that same year, Shulgin was an informal mentor to a group of graduate students in the Department of Chemistry of the University of California at San Francisco. One of these students, Merrie Kleinman, told him of the experience that she and two of her friends had had with MDMA[5] First synthesized in 1912, no one had previously reported its psychoactivity. Intrigued, Shulgin made up a batch of the drug and took 100 mg by mouth. In *PiHKAL*, he tells us of his very first experience with MDMA.

> I found it unlike anything I had taken before. It was not a psychedelic in the
> visual or interpretive sense, but the lightness and warmth of the psychedelic
> was present and quite remarkable. . . . My mood was light, happy, but with an
> underlying conviction that something significant was about to happen. . . . My
> usually poor vision was sharpened. I saw details in the distance that I could not
> normally see. After the peak experience had passed, my major state was one
> of deep relaxation. I felt that I could talk about personal subjects with special
> clarity.[6]

As was his custom, Shulgin soon shared MDMA with his friends and collected their comments. One to whom the drug was given was Leo Zeff, a 65-year-old psychologist who, in his private practice, had long used LSD as an aid to psychotherapy. Zeff quickly became convinced of the "immeas-urable value of MDMA for trauma and grief counseling, for improving relationships, and for terminal illness." Although Dr. Zeff had been con-templating retirement, he instead became a kind of Johnny Appleseed for the drug, ultimately introducing several hundred fellow psychotherapists to its use.[7]

VARIATIONS ON PHENETHYLAMINE:
AMPHETAMINES, MESCALINE, MDMA

Any reader with an aversion to organic chemistry should feel free to skip the next two paragraphs. I want to talk a little bit about the chemical relationships between stimulants, hallucinogens, and MDMA. In chapter 4, we met phenylethylamine (PEA), a chemical found in our brains. The phenyl group consists of six carbon atoms arranged in a circle. To this ring is attached a side chain consisting of two carbon atoms (an ethyl group) ending in an amine: phenyl-CH_2-CH_2-NH_2. If we now add a methyl group (CH_3) to the carbon adjacent to the amine, we have amphetamine. Add an additional methyl group to the amine of amphetamine and we have methamphetamine. As we learned in chapter 3, both amphetamine and methamphetamine are powerful stimulants.

If we number the six carbon atoms of the phenyl ring 1 through 6, we have a convenient way of expressing where substitutions have been made. The side chain of PEA is at the number 1 position. By adding methoxy groups (OCH_3) at the 3, 4, and 5 positions, we profoundly alter the pharmacological properties of PEA. Thus, 3, 4, 5-trimethoxyphenylethylamine is mescaline, the classical hallucinogen discussed in chapter 7. Alternatively, if the number 3 and 4 carbon atoms of the phenyl ring of methamphetamine are joined by a bridge consisting of two oxygen atoms separated by a carbon atom (methylenedioxy), we have methylenedioxymethamphetamine, MDMA.

Given MDMA's chemical relationship to methamphetamine, it is not surprising that it shares some of that drug's properties; both, for example, can increase blood pressure and heart rate. And, with MDMA's substitutions on the phenyl ring, elements of hallucinogenic activity might be expected. Indeed, MDMA is often classified as a hallucinogen. But recall Shulgin's thoughts on his first experience with the drug: "It was not a psychedelic in the visual or interpretive sense . . ."

Some who believe that MDMA is unique, neither a stimulant nor a hallucinogen, have suggested unique names. Ralph Metzner, a colleague of Timothy Leary and a prolific author on matters psychedelic, favored *empathogen*, an inducer of empathy, sensitivity to the thoughts and feelings of another.[8] Not all were enamored of the term. David Nichols, arguing that MDMA did more than generate empathy, coined the term *entactogen*. Thus, MDMA enables a patient to uncover and deal with painful emotional issues that are not ordinarily accessible.[9] It is Dr. Nichols, being both a pharmacologist and a skilled synthetic chemist, who has provided chemically pure MDMA to virtually all of the FDA-approved studies conducted over the past three decades. In recreational use, MDMA has been called at various times *Molly*, *The Luv Drug* (the same name has been given to MDMA's close chemical relative, MDA, methylenedioxyamphetamine), or, in England, *Mandy*. Most enduring has been *Ecstasy*, a term most often attributed to Michael Clegg, the leading supplier of MDMA prior to its being declared illegal.[10]

PSYCHOTHERAPISTS, RECREATIONAL USE, AND SCHEDULE I

Beginning in 1977, largely due to the proselytism of Leo Zeff, MDMA quickly became established as a useful aid to psychotherapy. The first scientific account of MDMA's efficacy in this regard was published in a 1978 book chapter by Alexander Shulgin and David Nichols.[11] Based on the experiences of multiple therapists with the drug, they stated that MDMA "evoked an easily controlled altered state of consciousness, with emotional and sensual overtones." The only adverse effects noted were occasional anxiety and transient effects on heart rate and blood pressure. However, at the same time, MDMA was becoming a popular recreational drug with demand being met by persons such as Michael Clegg. At its peak, the Clegg laboratory in California was said to be turning out 2 million doses of MDMA every month; half of those ended up in Dallas.[12]

One who took notice was Texas senator Lloyd Bentsen, who in May 1984 called upon the Drug Enforcement Administration (DEA) to issue an emergency ban on MDMA. The DEA listened and, on May 31, 1984, it was announced in the Federal Register that is was planning to place MDMA in Schedule I within 30 days. A hearing was requested to "determine the future status of the drug, such as to whether it should be placed in Schedule I."[13]

Four hearings took place in 1985. They were presided over by Francis Young, an Administrative Law Judge of the DEA. Psychotherapists expressed their belief that MDMA was a safe and effective drug when used in a medical setting as an adjunct to psychotherapy. Equally vocal were those who saw Ecstasy as a threat to society. Legalization, they believed, would send "the wrong message," especially to the young.

On May 22, 1986, Judge Young recommended that MDMA be placed in Schedule III. Thus, MDMA would join drugs such as ketamine and codeine. These are characterized as having (a) a potential for abuse less than the drugs of Schedules I and II, (b) a currently accepted medical use in treatment in the United States, and (c) may lead to minimal physical or high psychological dependence. It appeared that MDMA had escaped the strictures of Schedule I and would soon become available for medical use. It was not to be. In October 1986, Judge Young was overruled by the head of the DEA and, the following month, MDMA was placed in Schedule I. After legal skirmishes that lasted nearly 2 years, the Schedule I assignment was made permanent and remains in effect today.[14] Federal and state penalties for possession or sale of MDMA vary depending upon the amount of drug involved. In New York State, for example, mere possession of less than 25 mg of MDMA calls for a sentence of up to 1 year in prison. (Recall that Alexander Shulgin's initial dose was 100 mg.)

POSTTRAUMATIC STRESS DISORDER
AND THE CRUSADE OF DR. DOBLIN

The struggle to remove MDMA from Schedule I and to make it available for use as an adjunct to psychotherapy has been led for more than three decades by Rick Doblin, PhD, a man who is both scientist and activist. In 1986, the year that MDMA was declared illegal, Doblin founded the Multidisciplinary Association for Psychedelic Studies (MAPS), a non-profit organization with the broad goal of "raising awareness and understanding of psychedelics." Since then, MAPS has funded studies in this country and abroad on drugs such as LSD, psilocybin, ayahuasca, ibogaine, and ketamine for conditions ranging from drug and alcohol abuse to terminal illness to the anxiety of autistic adults. However, MAPS recently stated that "Our highest priority project is funding clinical trials of MDMA as a tool to assist psychotherapy for the treatment of post-traumatic stress disorder."[15]

The traumatic events that led to PTSD come in various forms: childhood abuse, sexual assault, refugee status, and wartime experiences are among the most common. The resulting stress can take many forms as well, but anxiety is a nearly universal feature. Nightmares and sleeplessness often occur. The risk of suicide is increased.

Let us begin with a woman named Sarah.[16] As a child, her father abused the whole family, but Sarah was often singled out. The winter Sarah was 11, she brought in the wrong wood for the fireplace, so her father locked her in the family's unfinished concrete basement. Her meals were brought to the top of the stairs. It was a freezing Christmas in Pennsylvania. The memory of this and other terrors remained with her 30 years later as an educated mother of a young son. Her heart would race at the sound of a clicking door or the barking of a dog, and she had difficulty in concentrating in social situations. Anxiety was a constant companion. Sarah could sleep only with windows and doors open to avoid a fear of being trapped.

It is likely that soldiers have suffered from what we now call post-traumatic stress disorder (PTSD) for as long as there has been war, but the term did not enter the psychiatric lexicon until 1980 in the third edition of *The Diagnostic and Statistical Manual of Mental Disorders* of the American Psychiatric Association. In World War I it was called shell shock. Veterans of World War II were said to suffer from battle fatigue. For those who had served in Vietnam, it was simply post-Vietnam syndrome. In a report from the Congressional Budget Office published in 2013, it was estimated that PTSD was present in 20% of the veterans of our wars in Iraq and Afghanistan. What follows is the account provided by one of them.

> It's been almost a year since my trauma, and even going to therapy and getting help for all my symptoms it is a long road. I'm basically having to re-learn how to control my emotions, my mouth, my anger, my *everything*. It's made it so I don't really know who I am or how I feel. Someone will just say, "How are you?" and I feel dumb for having to answer, "I don't know." Things run through my head like: I feel like a piece of shit for not being able to move on. Or I feel like it's basically like being an adult with the brain of a two-year-old with all the adult fears that drive everything. But finding the words to express this is so difficult for me now. I long for normalcy, for the person I used to be. Where I once saw myself as a confident, intelligent, out-going, all-together person, it now feels like a circus in my head. I don't understand myself any longer. Everything can overwhelm me. Thankfully, I am learning now how to cope and control it but honestly, I just am looking forward for this nightmare to end.[17]

Current treatment for PTSD is centered on one or another form of psychotherapy. The program currently favored by the Veterans Administration is prolonged exposure therapy, in which veterans over the course of 8–15 weekly sessions are guided in revisiting the traumatic memory and are repeatedly confronted with situations that mimic their traumatic event.[18] Although a number of medications have been used off-label, only two have received FDA approval. These are paroxetine (Paxil) and sertraline (Zoloft). Both are selective serotonin reuptake inhibitors (SSRIs), members of a family used very widely for both anxiety and depression. While few question the value of psychotherapy, there is no consensus as to what is the most effective form. The relative lack of efficacy of today's treatment for PTSD—some put the figure at no better than 20%—combined with the adverse effects connected with the use of SSRIs make it clear, at least to persons such as Rick Doblin, that MDMA is an attractive candidate for investigation. Some may find it remarkable that the Veterans Administration, which spends a substantial amount of money each year treating PTSD, has expressed an interest in MDMA but an unwillingness to fund research.

GEORGE RICAURTE AND "AN OUTRAGEOUS SCANDAL"

The route by which a drug goes from being an interesting molecule in the hands of a chemist such as Alexander Shulgin to a therapeutic agent is long and challenging. The overseer of that route is the FDA, which must grant its approval at each stage of the process. For MDMA, this began with toxicity studies in animals completed in 1987. This was followed in 1994 by a double blind, placebo-controlled study of MDMA in healthy volunteers; no significant adverse effects were noted. The first Phase 2 study to specifically address the efficacy of MDMA for PTSD was begun in Spain in 2000 under the direction of Jose Carlos Bouso. Protocol development, therapist training, and financial support were provided by MAPS. The subjects were six women who had been the victims of sexual assault. Initial results were promising, and the plan was to include 29 women. Unfortunately, following what Dr. Bouso called "political pressure," the study was terminated by the Madrid Anti-Drug Authority.[19]

In 2001, while the Spanish study was ongoing, Doblin received FDA approval for a similar Phase 2 investigation to be conducted in the United States. But several years would pass before recruitment of subjects could begin. The reason was that a serious roadblock had been thrown up by a publication which appeared on September 27, 2002. The senior author was George Ricaurte of the Department of Neurology of the Johns Hopkins University School of Medicine. The title of Ricaurte's paper tells the story: "Severe Dopaminergic Neurotoxicity After a Common Recreational Dose of MDMA ('Ecstasy')."[20] Most ominous was the suggestion by Ricaurte that persons exposed to MDMA would be at higher risk of Parkinson's disease "either as young adults or later in life." It has long been known that Parkinson's disease is caused by loss of dopaminergic neurons in a specific area of the brain related to motor function.

It appeared that the Ricaurte paper would put an end to Doblin's hopes for MDMA as an adjunct to psychotherapy. Furthermore, Ricaurte's dire warnings were used to aid passage on April 30, 2003, of the Illicit Drug Anti-Proliferation Act.[21] An earlier version had been called the RAVE (Reducing Americans' Vulnerability to Ecstasy) Act. The DEA hailed the modified act as a means to prosecute the promoters of any event where Ecstasy was used. But fortune smiled on Doblin in an odd way. On September 12, 2003, just short of 1 year after the appearance of the original report, a retraction was issued by Dr. Ricaurte.[22] Because of a mislabeled container, his monkeys had been treated, not with MDMA, but with methamphetamine. Leslie Iversen, a distinguished British pharmacologist and, most recently, visiting professor of neuropharmacology at the University of Oxford, characterized the episode as "an outrageous scandal."[23] An editorial in the international science magazine *Nature* called it "one of the most bizarre episodes in the history of drug research."[24]

THE CRUSADE GOES ON

In 2004, 3 years after its original approval, subjects began to be enrolled in the MAPS-funded study of the use of MDMA as an adjunct to psychotherapy for PTSD. The investigator was Michael Mithoefer, MD, a Charleston, South Carolina, psychiatrist in private practice. In conjunction with psychothera-peutic sessions, 12 participants received MDMA on two or three occasions while 8 others received an inactive placebo. All participants were classi-fied as being treatment resistant; that is, they had not responded to pre-vious administration of drugs or psychotherapy. One of those receiving MDMA was Sarah, the woman we met earlier in this chapter who had been terrorized as a child. PTSD during and after treatment was assessed with a standard rating scale. After 2 months, it was found that 10 of the 12 who had received MDMA no longer met the criteria for PTSD; in the pla-cebo group, improvement was limited to just 2 of 8. None of those treated with MDMA experienced adverse effects.[25] Sarah was one of those who improved significantly.

Doblin's crusade is not yet completed, but his goal is in sight. Mithoefer's findings, together with results from a similar study conducted in Switzerland under MAPS sponsorship, provided sufficient evidence of benefit coupled with minimal risk that the FDA permitted further Phase 2 studies to be conducted.[26] Thus, four other double-blind trials were completed by 2016 in the United States, Switzerland, Israel, and Canada, again with positive results. A study by Dr. Mithoefer's group yielded positive results in 26 vet-erans, police, and firefighters suffering from PTSD.[27] Overall, 2 months after the second experimental session, PTSD was no longer present in 53% of those treated with MDMA, a result far superior to that of psychotherapy alone. One year after the last MDMA session, 67% of the subjects no longer qualified for a diagnosis of PTSD.

The anti-anxiety effect of MDMA surely plays a role in its efficacy in treating PTSD. I am unaware of studies which explore the possible efficacy of MDMA in generalized anxiety disorder, but, in studies begun in 2014, promising results have been obtained in autistic adults who suffer from severe social anxiety.[28]

The final testing, referred to as Phase 3, will take the form of two double-blind trials in 200 to 300 PTSD patients. And, if all goes according to Doblin's hopes and expectations and previous positive results are replicated, it is expected that a New Drug Application (IND) will be approved by the FDA sometime in 2021, thus placing MDMA in the hands of specially trained psychotherapists for the treatment of PTSD. Thirty-five years will have passed since Doblin's founding of MAPS.

ECSTASY AS A DRUG OF ABUSE

Now let us turn from the potential therapeutic value of MDMA to its use as a recreational drug or, as others would characterize it, a drug of abuse. *Rave* is a word that entered the English language more than four centuries ago to describe wild, overly enthusiastic, or irrational talk. More recently, *rave* has taken on the additional meaning of an all-night dance party accompanied by electronic music and psychoactive drugs; MDMA is often one of the ingredients. Any attempt to define the medical risks associated with the use of MDMA must acknowledge the differences between the controlled setting of the psychotherapist's couch and the environment of a rave.

In the more than four decades which have passed since Alexander Shulgin introduced Leo Zeff to MDMA, a consistent picture of the hazards of the use of MDMA as an adjunct to psychotherapy has emerged. The conclusion drawn today is that the risks are minimal in mentally and physically healthy individuals. That caveat, "mentally and physically healthy," must be stated because, for example, while transient sympathomimetic effects such as increased heart rate and blood pressure may be harmless in most, they are a significant hazard when heart disease is present. Likewise, it is well established that in some persons latent psychiatric problems may emerge following the administration of MDMA. Best documented is an exacerbation of depression.[29] For these reasons, all who enter into MAPS-sponsored studies of PTSD are carefully screened to eliminate those persons with pre-existing medical or psychiatric conditions such as psychosis or bipolar disorder, though people suffering from depression can be enrolled in studies.

Upon leaving the world of carefully controlled therapeutic tests of efficacy of MDMA in treating PTSD and entering the environment of a rave or other venue in which Ecstasy is used, we encounter much greater uncertainty. In the therapeutic setting, a modest dose is given on a few occasions separated in time. In contrast, illicit use may involve much higher doses taken on multiple occasions by persons of uncertain medical and psychiatric predisposition. Adding to the ambiguity is the sometimes uncertain chemical identity of Ecstasy and the general failure to determine blood or urine levels of MDMA following a toxic episode.

Unlike the opiates, Ecstasy rarely kills its users. Most of the deaths reliably attributed to Ecstasy have resulted from hyperthermia, a body temperature of greater than 104°F. Untreated, hyperthermia can rapidly lead to nausea and vomiting, confusion, convulsions, and coma. There may be irreversible damage to liver, kidneys, and the brain. Ecstasy-related hyperthermia is a form of exertional heat stroke brought on by strenuous dancing in the hot environment of a rave. While there is no question that death may result from hyperthermia, the two most famous fatalities associated with Ecstasy were, ironically, likely the result of attempts to avoid hyperthermia.

In 1995, Anna Wood was a teenager growing up in a suburb of Sydney, Australia. On the evening of October 21, she and her friends bought tablets of Ecstasy and entered a rave at a club in downtown Sydney. At 5 a.m. the next morning, after a night of dancing, Anna began to vomit. By 10 a.m., she fell into unconsciousness. Two days later, Anna died; she was 15 years of age.[30] Less than a month after Anna's death, an English girl named Leah Betts swallowed an Ecstasy tablet with friends and, 4 hours later, she lost consciousness. Leah died 5 days later; she had entered her 18th year of life just 2 weeks earlier.[31]

Advice given to avoid hyperthermia is to drink plenty of water, thus replacing the electrolytes lost in sweat during prolonged, vigorous dancing. In Australia, the public health message was "Water is an antidote to dancing." Both Anna and Leah took that advice. Leah drank nearly 3 gallons of water after taking Ecstasy. Anna was said to have drunk fluids throughout her night of dancing. Upon completion of autopsies, it was concluded that both Leah and Anna had died as a result of water intoxication, leading to swelling of the brain. In a condition known as hyponatremia, blood levels of sodium fall to life-threatening levels. This is brought about by the dilution of bodily fluids by excess water intake. In addition, it is likely that MDMA exacerbates the problem by diminishing the loss of water through urination

Tragic as is the death of anyone, especially a young person, as a consequence of drug use, the number of fatalities due to MDMA or Ecstasy is vanishingly small compared with the number directly attributable to opiates or tobacco. (We must remind ourselves that smoking kills more Americans than car crashes, murder, and drugs combined.) Nonetheless, continued widespread illicit use of MDMA carries with it the possibility of long-term adverse effects. Perhaps most troubling were reports in the first decade of this century which suggested that subtle deficits in memory may occur and persist long after use of MDMA or Ecstasy has stopped.[32,33,34,35] Reassuringly, a subsequent investigation conducted at the Harvard Medical School and funded by the FDA, after correcting for many of the design deficiencies of the earlier work, failed to replicate these findings.[36] But the issue has not gone away. A report published in 2014 by a group at London Metropolitan University concluded with these words: " . . . the prognosis for the current generation of ecstasy users is a major cause for concern."[37]

NO DEFINITIVE ANSWERS

Will MDMA in combination with psychotherapy prove to be a cure for many suffering the effects of PTSD and other psychiatric disorders? Will the pleasures of recreational and perhaps even medical use of MDMA come at the price of memory deficits in the future? Will there come a time, as occurred with marijuana, that some will call for the legalization of MDMA for recreational use? No definitive answers to these questions can be provided at this time.

NOTES

1. Tanner-Smith EE (2006) Pharmacological content of tablets sold as "ecstasy": Results from an online testing service. *Drug Alcohol Depend* 83(3):247–254.
2. Shulgin S, Shulgin A (1991) *PiHKAL: A Chemical Love Story*. Berkeley, CA: Transform Press.
3. Shulgin S, Shulgin A (1997) *TiHKAL: The Continuation*. Berkeley, CA: Transform Press.
4. Boal M (2004) The agony and ecstasy of Alexander Shulgin. *Playboy*. March.
5. Shulgin S, Shulgin A (1991) *PiHKAL: A Chemical Love Story*. Berkeley, CA: Transform Press.
6. Shulgin S, Shulgin A (1991) *PiHKAL: A Chemical Love Story*. Berkeley, CA: Transform Press.
7. Shulgin S, Shulgin A (1991) *PiHKAL: A Chemical Love Story*. Berkeley, CA: Transform Press.
8. Adamson S (1986) *Through the Gateway of the Heart: Accounts of Experiences With MDMA and Other Empathogenic Substances*. San Francisco: Four Trees Publications.
9. Nichols DE (1986) Differences between the mechanisms of action of MDMA, MBDB, and the classical hallucinogens. Identification of a new therapeutic class: Entactogens. *J Psychoact. Drugs* 18:305–313.
10. Doblin R (2019) Personal communication.
11. Shulgin AT, Nichols DE (1978) Characterization of three new psychotomimetics. In *The Psychopharmacology of Hallucinogens*, R Stillman, R Willete, Eds. New York: Pergamon Press.

12. Doblin R (2019) Personal communication.

13. Anonymous (1985) U.S. will ban "Ecstasy," a hallucinogenic drug. *New York Times*, June 1.

14. Lawn JC (1986) Schedules of controlled substances: Scheduling of 3,4-methylenedioxymethamphetamine (MDMA) into Schedule I. *Federal Register* 51:36552–36560.

15. Multidisciplinary Association for Psychedelic Studies (MAPS) (2018) https://maps.org

16. Winter, JL (2011) Can a single pill change your life? *O, The Oprah Magazine*, March. (Full disclosure: JL Winter is my daughter, Jessica.)

17. Military with PTSD (2018) What does PTSD feel like? https://www.militarywithptsd.org/

18. Eftekhari A, Ruzek JI, Crowley JJ, Rosen CS, Greenbaum MA, Karlin BE (2013) Effectiveness of national implementation of prolonged exposure therapy in Veterans Affairs care. *JAMA Psychiatry* 70(9):949–955.

19. Bouso JC, Doblin R, Farre M, Alcazar MA, Gomez-Jarabo G (2008) MDMA-assisted psychotherapy using low doses in a small sample of women with chronic posttraumatic stress disorder. *J Psychoactive Drugs* 40(3):225–236.

20. Ricaurte GA, Yuan J, Hatzidimitriou G, Cord BJ, McCann UD (2002) Severe dopaminergic neurotoxicity in primates after a common recreational dose of MDMA (Ecstasy). *Science* 297:2260–2263.

21. Congress of the United States (2003–2004) S.226—Illicit Drug Anti-Proliferation Act of 2003. https://www.congress.gov/bill/108th-congress/senate-bill/226

22. Ricaurte GA, Yuan J, Hatzidimitriou G, Cord BJ, McCann UD. (2003) Retraction.

23. Wahl R (2003) Retracted Ecstasy paper "an outrageous scandal." *The Scientist* 301:1479.

24. Anonymous (2003) Ecstasy's after-effects. *Nature* 425(223) issue 6925, September 18.

25. Mithoefer MC, Wagner MT, Mithoefer AT, Jerome L, Doblin R (2011) The safety and efficacy of {+/-}3,4-methylenedioxymethamphetamine-assisted psychotherapy in subjects with chronic, treatment-resistant posttraumatic stress disorder: The first randomized controlled pilot study. *J Psychopharmacol* 25(4):439–452.

26. Feduccia AA, Holland J, Mithoefer MC (2018) Progress and promise for the MDMA drug development program. *Psychopharmacology* 235(2):561–571.

27. Mithoefer MC, Mithoefer AT, Feduccia AA, Jerome L, Wagner M, Wymer J, Holland J, Hamilton S, Yazar-Klosinski B, Emerson A, Doblin R (2018) 3,4-methylenedioxymethamphetamine (MDMA)-assisted psychotherapy for posttraumatic stress disorder in military veterans, firefighters, and police officers: a randomized, double-blind, dose-response, phase 2 clinical trial. *Lancet Psychiatry* 5(6):486–497.

28. Danforth AL, Grob CS, Struble C, Feduccia AA, Walker N, Jerome L, Yazar-Klosinki B, Emerson A (2018) Reduction in social anxiety after MDMA-assisted psychotherapy with autistic adults: A randomized, double-blind, placebo-controlled pilot study. *Psychopharmacology* 235(11):3137–3148.

29. Taurah L, Chandler C, Sanders G (2014) Depression, impulsiveness, and memory in past and present polydrug users of 3,4-methylenedioxymethamphetamine (MDMA, ecstasy). Psychopharmacology 231:737–751.

30. Erowid MDMA Vaults (1995) Water Intoxication Death. https://erowid.org/chemicals/mdma/mdma_health5.shtml

31. Laurance J (1995) *The Times*. Leah Betts dies of drinking water to counter drug's effect. www.urban75.com/Drugs/drugxtc1.html
32. Lyvers M (2006) Recreational use and the neurotoxic potential of MDMA. *Drug Alc Review* 25:269–276.
33. Gouzoulis-Mayfrank E, Daumann J (2006) Neurotoxicity of MDMA in humans: How strong is the evidence for persistent brain damage? *Addiction* 101:348–361.
34. Kalechstein AD, De La Garza R, Mahoney JJ, Fantegrossi WE, Newton TF (2007) MDMA use and neurocognition: A meta-analytic review. *Psychopharmacology* 189:531–537.
35. Rogers G, Elston J, Garside R, Roome C, Younger P (2009) The harmful health effects of recreational ecstasy. *Health Technol Assess* 13(6):1–315.
36. Halpern JH, Sherwood AR, Hudson JI, Gruber S, Kozin D, Pope HG Jr (2011) Residual neurocognitive features of long-term ecstasy users with minimal exposure to other drugs. *Addiction* 106(4):777–786.
37. Taurah L, Chandler C, Sanders G (2014) Depression, impulsiveness, and memory in past and present polydrug users of 3,4-methylenedioxymethamphetamine (MDMA, ecstasy). Psychopharmacology 231:737–751.

CHAPTER 9

cᎧᴐ

Pharmacological Puritanism
and the War on Drugs

All the King's Horses and All the King's Men . . .

H. L. Mencken, arguably the leading satirist of the 20th century, said that American puritanism is characterized by the haunting fear that someone, somewhere, may be happy.[1] If the source of that happiness is a drug, we might call it pharmacological puritanism. Followers of that faith abound, but I will mention just few. "There's no such thing as recreational drug use" were the words of William Weld, head of the criminal division of the Attorney General's office in 1988.[2] A year later, in the midst of a cocaine epidemic, William Bennett, the first director of the Office of National Drug Control Policy (ONDCP) under President George H. W. Bush, expressed dual goals. The first was to construct 95,000 more federal prison cells for drug abusers and the second to make Washington, D.C., a drug-free city. He believed that calls for legalization of any psychoactive drug to be "morally scandalous."[3] John Walters, director of the ONDCP during George W. Bush's tenure as president, believed that religion is the answer to drug abuse. Lest we think that pharmacological puritanism is a dying faith, we need only recall Attorney General Jeff Sessions' comment in 2016 that "Good people don't smoke marijuana."[4] It does make me wonder where, on the good–bad spectrum, lie the tens of millions of Americans who live in states and in the District of Columbia where marijuana is legal for recreational use.

Our Love Affair with Drugs: The History, the Science, the Politics. Jerrold Winter, Oxford University Press (2020). © Jerrold Winter.
DOI: 10.1093/oso/9780190051464.001.0001

Among the general population, pharmacological puritanism appears to be uncommon. A survey of American college students found that the prime motives for drug use were to help with concentration, to increase alertness, and to get high.[5] From the United Kingdom, David Nutt, chairman of the Department of Neuropsychopharmacology at Imperial College London, put it this way: "Drugs are taken for pleasure."[6] Whatever their numbers today or in the past, it is believers in pharmacological puritanism, with the absolutism which accompanies that faith, who are major contributors to the failure of our most recent war on drugs, now nearly a half-century old.

In some religions, in some parts of the world, apostasy, renunciation of the faith, is a sin punishable by death. It appears that pharmacological puritanism is more forgiving. Earlier I mentioned William Weld's statement that "there is no such thing as recreational drug use." In April 2018, it was announced that Mr. Weld had joined the board of advisors of Acreage Holdings, a multistate company devoted to the cultivation, processing, and selling of cannabis products. He was joined on the board by John Boehner, a former congressman from Ohio and speaker of the United States House of Representatives from 2011 to 2015, who previously had been "unalterably opposed" to the legalization of marijuana. Acreage Holdings moto is "Leading the Way to Safe Cannabis for Everyone."

DEFINING DRUG ABUSE

What we call a war on drugs might more properly be declared a war on drug abuse. And there we encounter our first problem. Drug abuse is a social construct reflecting deviation from accepted social, religious, or medical customs. For example, treatment of postsurgical or cancer pain to the point of tolerance and physical dependence on morphine or fentanyl does not legally or socially make one a drug abuser. Use of the same amount of fentanyl or morphine in a nonmedical setting will mark a person as an addict.

Turning to social customs, the situation is murkier yet. These customs are often influenced to a significant degree by religious beliefs. These are handed down by God and thus not susceptible to rational analysis or refutation. For example, Rastifarianism is a religious movement among black Jamaicans that includes the ritualistic use of marijuana, yet even possession of marijuana remains illegal under federal law in the United States. In chapter 7, we learned of the legally sanctioned sacramental use of the hallucinogens psilocybin and mescaline, both Schedule I drugs, by members of indigenous religious groups. When, during the winter of 1833 in Kirtland, Ohio, Joseph Smith, founder of the Mormon religion, had a conversation with God, he was told that "inasmuch as any man drinketh wine or strong drink among you, behold it is not good."[7] The confusion which can arise was cinematically illustrated by the Cohen brothers in their film *Burn After Reading*. Osbourne Cox, a CIA analyst, is told by his superior that he is being relieved of his duties. Cox asks why, and a fellow agent, Peck, interjects, "You have a drinking problem." Cox replies, "I have a drinking problem? Fuck you, Peck, you're a Mormon. Next to you, we all have a drinking problem." Thus, it is circumstance, not pharmacology or even toxicology, that defines drug abuse.

If we are to fight a war on drugs, it would be a good idea to define what "success" will look like. For the pharmacological puritan, victory must be total: a United States devoid of psychoactive drugs, with the exception, of course, of nicotine and alcohol. American puritans are not alone. In 1998, the United Nations hosted a General Assembly Special Session under the official slogan: "A Drug-Free World: We Can Do It."[8] Nonpuritanical goals are more modest: (1) to maximize the pleasure derived from drugs, with pleasure defined in very broad terms to include, for example, relief of anxiety or enhancement of performance, and (2) to minimize the harm done by these drugs. In other words, for each drug under consideration, to optimize the benefit–risk ratio. Our experience over the past century has shown that pursuit of a country or a world free of psychoactive drugs is unattainable, undesirable, and immensely harmful and expensive.

THE ROOTS OF THE WAR ON DRUGS

It is true that the phrase "war on drugs" is most often associated with Richard Nixon beginning in the late 1960s, but the origins of that war go back much further. The law was often a weapon in that war. As has been pointed out by George Fisher, professor of law at Stanford University, drug laws initially appeared at the community and state levels.[9] The first, in 1875, came from the San Francisco Board of Supervisors who made it a misdemeanor to visit an opium den. Professor Fisher points out that the intent of the law was not to deny the use of opium to Chinese but, instead, in the words in 1875 of the *San Francisco Chronicle*, to suppress "opium-smoking establishments run by the Chinese for exclusive use by white men and women of respectable parentage." Echoing such thoughts more than a century later are those who suggest that our current opioid epidemic became a national concern only when opioid use escaped the minority populations of our inner cities and threatened the lives of young white America. In any event, the years ending the 19th century and early into the 20th saw local and state laws passed which criminalized the use of opium, cocaine, and marijuana.

The federal government entered the legal fray in 1909 by prohibiting the importation of opium for any but medicinal purposes. The Harrison Narcotic Act of 1914 added cocaine-containing coca leaves to the prohibited list. In the years that followed, the federal farms we discussed in chapter 2 were created "for the confinement and treatment of persons addicted to the use of habit-forming narcotic drugs." The Bureau of Narcotics, precursor to today's Drug Enforcement Administration, was formed in 1930. Under the leadership of Harry Anslinger, the first commissioner of the Federal Bureau of Narcotics whom we met in chapter 3, the Marijuana Tax Act was passed in 1937. It required the registration of "Any person who deals in, dispenses, or gives away marijuana . . . "[10]

In a choice piece of pharmacological irony, it was Timothy Leary who was responsible for repeal of the Marijuana Tax Act.[11] In December 1965, Leary and his two teenage children were in Texas returning from a vacation in Mexico when border agents discovered marijuana in their car. Leary was arrested, charged under the 1937 Act, and 3 months later sentenced to 30 years in prison and fined $30,000. His appeal of that arrest reached the Supreme Court of the United States in 1969. Leary's conviction was overturned on the grounds that his Fifth Amendment rights against self-incrimination had been violated. In complying with the Tax Act, he incriminated himself as a user of marijuana, a crime in Texas punishable by imprisonment. The next year, the Act was repealed and replaced with the Comprehensive Drug Abuse Prevention and Control Act, which established drug Schedules and placed marijuana in Schedule I.

A recurring pharmacological fault in laws designed to inhibit drug abuse is failure to discriminate between drugs. Thus, cocaine, opioids, and cannabis were lumped together with the label of "narcotic drugs." As we have seen in the preceding chapters, each drug class and each drug within a class has its own set of benefits and hazards. Thus, to place in the same legal category drugs as disparate as heroin, with its highly significant potential for causing death following overdose, and a relatively benign drug such as marijuana, is to invite frustration and failure.

RICHARD NIXON'S WAR ON DRUGS

Some may find it curious that Richard Nixon, a man alleged to have been fond of alcohol, sometimes in excessive quantities, should today be identified so closely with the war on drugs. (Often we hear the phrase "drugs and alcohol" as if alcohol were not a perfectly proper drug, and a particularly dangerous one at that.) On June 17, 1971, Nixon said that "America's public enemy number one is drug abuse. In order to fight and defeat this enemy, it is necessary to wage a new, all-out offensive."[12] The explanation for this fervor appears to have had little to do with drugs per se but instead with Nixon's visceral dislike of African Americans, hippies, and those protesting the Vietnam war.

Racism, of course, has had a long history in efforts to make certain drugs illegal. For more than a century, the tabloid press has delighted in stories of immigrant Mexicans made mad by marijuana, cocaine-crazed blacks attacking white women, and, more benignly, Chinese in opium-induced stupor. In Nixon's case, we have the word of John Ehrlichman, White House Counsel to Nixon, that blacks and war protestors were singled out for political reasons. In an interview with Dan Baum in 1994, an interview not revealed by Baum until 2016, Ehrlichman said the following:

> The Nixon campaign in 1968, and the Nixon White House after that, had two enemies: the antiwar left and black people. You understand what I'm saying? We knew we couldn't make it illegal to be either black or against the war, but by getting the public to associate the hippies with marijuana and blacks with heroin, and then criminalizing both heavily, we could disrupt those communities. We could arrest their leaders, raid their homes, break up their meetings, and vilify them night after night on the evening news. Did we know we were lying about the drugs? Of course we did.[13]

Whatever the effect that Nixon's war may have had on Vietnam protestors, that phase soon ended. In contrast, its disparities, and its adverse consequences, for African Americans have persisted for decades. In chapter 4, we had the example provided by cocaine. The Anti-Drug Abuse Act of 1986 mandated a 5-year prison sentence for possession of 5 grams of crack, the form of cocaine common among blacks, while possession of 100 times as much cocaine powder, the choice of whites, called for the same sentence.[14] According to the American Civil Liberties Union, 27 years after passage of the 1993 Rockefeller Drug Laws in New York State, more than 90% of persons incarcerated for drug offenses are African American or Latino. Between 1976 and 2006, there were 362,000 marijuana possession arrests in New York City.[15] Eighty-four percent of those arrested were either black or Latino despite a similar rate of marijuana use among whites. In 2016, the *Sarasota Herald-Tribune* reported that in nearly half the counties in Florida, blacks convicted of felony drug possession received jail time nearly double that given whites. African American women have been particularly hard hit. Between 1980 and 2009, the arrest rate for drug possession by women tripled. The vast majority of these women were poor and either black or Latino; 80% had children. Yet, 20 years ago, Barry McCaffrey, director of the Office of National Drug Control Policy in the administration of George W. Bush, said that "We can't incarcerate our way out of our drug problems."

THE END OF A NEW DAWN

During the presidency of Barack Obama, there were signs we might be heeding General McCaffrey's advice and plotting new tactics in our war on drugs. On May 11, 2010, the National Drug Control Strategy was released with the intent to pursue a more balanced approach with emphasis on prevention and treatment together with law enforcement. *The Lancet* called it "a new dawn."[16] That same year, the Fair Sentencing Act reduced the penalty disparity between crack and powder cocaine and eliminated mandatory minimum sentences. More significant changes had to do with marijuana. Early in the administration, the Office of the Attorney General advised US attorneys not to prosecute individuals providing medical marijuana in compliance with state laws despite continued federal illegality. In 2013, James Cole, Deputy Attorney General, extended that nonprosecution advice, in what came to be called the Cole memorandum, to include recreational marijuana.[17] Further protection for medical marijuana was provided by passage in December 2014 of the Rohrabacher-Farr amendment, which prohibits the use of federal funds to interfere with state medical marijuana laws.[18] President Obama commuted the sentences of nearly 600 nonviolent drug offenders. In 2015, the federal prison population declined for the first time in 33 years.

The hopes of those who foresaw a continued trend away from pharmacological puritanism were dashed in 2017 by President Donald Trump's appointment of Jeff Sessions as Attorney General of the United States. Oddly, given the increasing number of deaths from opioids and the nonlethality of marijuana, Sessions focused not on opioids but on marijuana by rescinding the Cole memo and calling for repeal of the Rohrabacher-Farr amendment. At that time, Tom Cotton, a Sessions supporter and senator from Arkansas, said that we suffer from "an under-incarceration problem."

Virtually all who have studied drug policy agree that our near half-century war on drugs has been a failure. But can we be more quantitative in assessing progress in the war? Let us use death from opioid overdose, an unequivocal endpoint, as our measure of success. Data are hard to come by before 1999, but a comparison of that year with 2017 is informative. In 1999, there were approximately 6,400 deaths attributed to heroin, morphine, and other opioids, a rate of 2.53 deaths for every 100,000 persons. The corresponding figures for 2017 were 53,332 deaths and a rate of 16.51 deaths per 100,000 persons.[19]

Pharmacological puritans who, like Sessions, advocate continuation, indeed, enhancement, of our previous efforts, including mass incarceration, remind me of a cartoon cited by Herbert Kleber, deputy director of the Office of National Drug Control Policy under William Bennett, the nation's first drug czar. The king is slamming his fist on the table, saying, "If all my horses and all my men can't put Humpty Dumpty together again, then what I need is more horses and more men." (Dr. Kleber left his position after just 2 years and expressed disappointment that the majority of funds available were directed at law enforcement rather than to treatment.)

We might wish to consider the words of Baruch Spinoza, a 17th-century Dutch philosopher:

> He who seeks to regulate everything by law is more likely to arouse vices than to reform them. It is best to grant what cannot be abolished, even though it be in itself harmful.[20]

THE EXAMPLE OF PORTUGAL

The polar opposite of pharmacological puritanism is the strict libertarian view that all psychoactive drugs should be completely legal. The United States is not ready now nor is it likely ever to be ready for that great leap, but a few countries have actually implemented some features of that approach. Portugal stands as the best-studied example.[21]

Beginning in the 1980s, Portugal found itself in the midst of a drug crisis. One estimate was that 10% of the country was using heroin with 1% of the entire population addicted to the drug. Largely due to the sharing of needles between addicts, the rate of HIV infection was the highest in Europe. After experiencing this epidemic for nearly two decades, a bold step was taken: revision of the penal code.

Though often touted as complete legalization of psychoactive drugs, this was not the case. Instead, there was decriminalization of possession and consumption of all illicit drugs. For example, anyone found with a drug such as heroin might simply be given a warning, hit with a small fine, or, if addiction was thought to be present, referred to a local commission consisting of a physician, a lawyer, and a social worker. The addict would then be advised regarding support services, harm reduction, and the availability of treatment programs.

Heroin use in Portugal has not been eliminated, but deaths from overdose, drug-related crime, and rates of incarceration have decreased significantly. By 2015, new cases of HIV infection fell by 95% from the record high 15 years earlier. A comparison of the number of deaths in 2015 from opioid overdose in Portugal and the United States is provocative: 63,600 in America, 27 in Portugal. But the United States has a much larger population, so death rate per million persons is more informative: 195 deaths per million in the United States, 2.6 per million in Portugal.

For those who favor a nonpuritanical approach to drug use, hope is engendered by recent events. For example, as discussed in chapter 3, our social and pharmacological experiment currently underway to legalize the use of marijuana for medical and recreational purposes will teach us much about how our society can address the promise and pitfalls presented by psychoactive drugs. Likewise informative will be the outcome of efforts described in the last chapter to make MDMA, a Schedule I drug, available for treatment of posttraumatic stress disorder, an all too often concomitant of service in our wars. With respect to marijuana, in 2018, California, Michigan, and Massachusetts joined the District of Columbia and the states of Alaska, Colorado, Maine, Nevada, Oregon, Vermont, Michigan, and Washington in legalizing recreational use. Thus, despite Attorney General Sessions's focus on a return to prosecution of all marijuana offenders (former Attorney General Eric Holder called it the "Sessions almost obsession"[22]), the trend toward pragmatic policies regarding at least some psychoactive drugs appears irreversible. Let us turn to our real problem, the opioid epidemic. How did it develop and what might a pragmatic approach to its amelioration, perhaps even its arrest, look like?

THE ROOTS OF THE OPIOID EPIDEMIC

In searching for causes of the opioid epidemic in the hope that we will find a remedy, two prime candidates have emerged. These are (1) corporate greed in the form of a drug called OxyContin and (2) the feckless and sometimes criminal prescribing habits of American physicians. Alas, the two are related.

As was noted in chapter 2, opium and its descendants, morphine and opioids, are unparalleled in their ability to relieve pain. However, in the

1970s, concerns began to be expressed in the medical community that these drugs were underutilized; too many Americans were living and dying in pain.[23] The concern was such that in 1995, the American Pain Society suggested that a fifth vital sign, pain, be added to the traditional four of heart rate, blood pressure, breathing, and body temperature.[24] Pain experienced before, during, and after treatment was to be assessed in every patient. Physicians were urged to use visual analog scales to rate pain from 1 to 10. Hospitals and medical care plans took to assessing physician performance based on the relief or elimination of pain. Primary among the drugs used to achieve these goals were the opioids.

Many physicians were, of course, aware of the warnings of the American Medical Association dating back to the 1940s regarding the dangers of addiction to opioids. But reassurance had come by way of a brief letter to the editor of *The New England Journal of Medicine* published on January 10, 1980.[25] There it was reported that among 11,882 hospitalized patients who had received an opioid, there were only four cases of addiction in those without a history of addiction. The authors' conclusion was that despite widespread use of opioids in hospitals, "the development of addiction is rare." Over the years that followed, this eight-line letter would be cited in the medical literature nearly a thousand times, with 70% citing it as evidence that addiction seldom occurs in patients treated with opioids. Physicians became much more liberal in their prescription of opioids both for the pain of terminal illness, a very good thing, and for the treatment of acute and chronic pain, a more problematic undertaking. One of the most popular drugs was oxycodone.

Oxycodone is a synthetic opioid with all of the properties of morphine and heroin. It is an effective pain reliever at moderate doses and can cause death by respiratory depression at higher doses. Tolerance and physical dependence will develop in all who take even moderate doses of oxycodone for an extended period of time. If stopped abruptly, a characteristic opioid withdrawal syndrome will be experienced. Some will find the effects of oxycodone to be highly rewarding, and they will become addicted.

Oxycodone is not a new drug. It was first synthesized more than a century ago. All of what I said in the preceding paragraph about oxycodone, including physical dependence and addiction, was known to the scientific and medical communities for decades. It is, after all, just another opioid whose chemical precursor is found in the opium poppy. How then did a modified form of oxycodone, OxyContin, become the poster child for corporate greed and medical malfeasance and, in achieving that status, play a major role in the opioid epidemic?[26]

One of the therapeutic principles observed in treating pain is to maintain an adequate level of relief at all times. Furthermore, one would prefer to have a drug which does not require administration at very short intervals. For example, oxycodone must be given every 4 hours. In OxyContin, Purdue Pharma, a Connecticut-based pharmaceutical company, had created a controlled-release form of oxycodone said to be effective for 12 hours. When this claim was found to be untrue, sales representatives ("detail men," though now many are women) for Purdue Pharma in their visits to doctors' offices advised physicians to increase the dose of OxyContin rather than to shorten the dosing interval. It was bad advice, but the reason for it is now clear. By continuing to endorse a longer dosing interval, Purdue Pharma buttressed their further claim, recklessly approved by the Food and Drug Administration (FDA), that OxyContin, compared with other opioids, was less likely to be abused or to lead to addiction. This was later found to be disastrously untrue.

Introduced in 1996, OxyContin was an immediate commercial success due in large measure to an aggressive marketing campaign directed at physicians and accompanied by advertising in medical journals. Opinion leaders in the medical community were recruited to present, at $500 per session, 15-minute presentations to fellow physicians, often over dinner provided by Purdue Pharma. Individual doctors enjoyed the hospitality of the company at warm weather resort properties where the nonaddictive virtues of OxyContin were extolled. Groups formed to promote the aggressive treatment of pain were funded in part by Purdue Pharma. The American Pain Society, which I mentioned earlier as the originator of "pain as the fifth vital sign," was one such organization.

By 2001, OxyContin accounted for half of all opioid prescriptions, 6 million of them at a cost of more than a billion dollars. At about the same time, reality began to raise its ugly head. Those prone to abuse or addiction soon learned that OxyContin tablets could be crushed and then snorted or injected to give an effect comparable to that of heroin. An added attraction was that an OxyContin tablet, as a sustained-release formulation, contained a lot of oxycodone. The 80 mg formulation was equivalent to as many as 32 tablets of Percocet, a combination of immediate-release oxycodone with acetaminophen.

On May 10, 2007, Purdue Pharma and three of its executives pleaded guilty in federal court to having "misbranded" OxyContin and in so doing misleading both the FDA and physicians as to the risk of abuse and addiction that the drug presented. The company was fined $600 million; an additional total of $35 million was paid by Purdue Pharma's chief lawyer, its president, and the former medical director. During its lifetime, sales of OxyContin were in excess of $40 billion. *Forbes* magazine estimated in 2015 that the heirs of the founders of Purdue Pharma, brothers Mortimer and Raymond Sackler, were worth a total of at least $14 billion, putting them among the 20 richest families in the United States. OxyContin had been very, very good to them. Amid a storm of lawsuits filed against Purdue Pharma, drug distributors, and pharmacy chains, the company announced in February 2018 that it would cut its sales force in half and stop marketing OxyContin in the United States.

Lest we believe that the Purdue Pharma playbook for promotion of opioid sales passed into history with the legal settlements in 2007, we should consider another opioid, fentanyl, and its marketing by Insys Therapeutics, an Arizona-based drug house. In 2012, Insys gained FDA approval for a form of fentanyl, trade name Subsys, to be sprayed under the tongue for the treatment of what is called breakthrough pain. An example is pain that can arise spontaneously in cancer patients despite their maintenance on usually adequate doses of opioids.

In October 2017, John Kapoor, the billionaire founder of Insys, was charged with multiple crimes, including the authorization of kickbacks, under the Racketeer Influenced and Corrupt Organizations Act (RICO).[27] In March 2018, five New York physicians were indicted for engaging in a bribery and kickback scheme involving Subsys prescriptions.[28] The more prescriptions written, the greater the payments made directly to them from Insys Therapeutics. These payments were often disguised as honoraria for "educational" talks promoting the drug to fellow physicians. (A philanthropic note: Dr. Kapoor along with Mortimer and Raymond Sackler, the founders of Purdue Pharma, have been generous with their opioid-generated billions. This is witnessed by the University of Oxford's Sackler Library, Sackler Wings at the Metropolitan Museum of Art in New York City and at the Louvre Museum in Paris, the Sackler Centre for Arts Education at the Victoria and Albert Museum in London, and by bequests to countless other such institutions. John Kapoor has been less visible, but when a new building was dedicated in 2012 housing the School of Pharmacy and Pharmaceutical Sciences of the University at Buffalo, Dr. Kapoor's alma mater, it was given the name *John and Editha Kapoor Hall*. Alas, following the conviction of Dr. Kapoor on racketeering charges in 2019, it was announced that the building would be re-named.)

The relative contributions to the opioid epidemic made by unscrupulous marketing of opioids such as OxyContin and Subsys and by overzealous prescription of opioids by physicians will never be known. But these two factors can hardly be the whole story. After reaching a peak in 2010, opioid prescriptions had fallen 13% by 2015 and have continued to fall each year since. Despite this, opioid-related deaths have continued to rise in each year since 2010; a plateau, let alone a decrease, has not yet been seen. What is the explanation for this paradox? The answer, it seems to me, lies in two factors: (1) an ever-increasing supply of ever-more potent opioids and (2) an ever-increasing demand for opioids driven by multiple factors in American society.

CONTROLLING PRESCRIBING BY PHYSICIANS

There are only two sources of opioids for addicts: (a) illicit suppliers and (b) physicians and other health care providers allowed by law to prescribe opioids. To deal with prescribers, those of a puritanical bent might suggest that we eliminate opioids from the health care system. Such prohibition is totally unacceptable; opioids are much too valuable for the relief of pain and the comfort of the dying. Indeed, I am inclined to believe that only a masochist or one who has never suffered even moderate pain and the relief provided by opioids would suggest it. But we can attempt to control prescribing habits and the Centers for Disease Control and Prevention (CDC) has done exactly that.[29]

Issued in March 2016, CDC guidelines suggest that for pain expected to be of short duration, opioids for "three days or less will often be sufficient; more than seven days will rarely be needed." The general recommendations to address chronic pain include urine testing, prior to treatment, for any "controlled substances and illicit drugs" with the intent to identify prior drug use. If opioids are to be employed, the lowest possible dose is recommended with evaluation of benefit and harm every 3 months. For patients found to have an "opioid use disorder," treatment should be offered or arranged. Excluded from these guidelines were those persons being treated for cancer pain, palliative care, and end-of-life care. These are conditions in which generous use of opioids even to the point of physical dependence is accepted; opioid use disorder is not an issue.

The CDC's action was not without its critics. Among the more eloquent was Stephen Martin, a rural family physician in Massachusetts, and his colleagues, who called the guidelines "neat, plausible, and generally wrong."[30] He questioned why cancer pain was included in the guidelines while other chronic painful conditions such as sickle cell anemia, severe arthritis, spinal stenosis, inoperable kidney stones, and chronic pancreatitis were not. He pointed out that untreated chronic pain decreases life expectancy by 10 years and that the risk of suicide is doubled. Following the

OxyContin era, many took as accepted wisdom that opioid prescribing by physicians correlates directly with diversion and nonmedical use. However, Dr. Martin and his colleagues gave the example of the state of Colorado, where opioid prescribing is in the lowest fifth of all states yet in the highest fifth for nonmedical use.

In response to the CDC guidelines, many physicians sharply reduced the amount of opioids prescribed. Some practices proudly announced that opioids would no longer be used at all. An unintended consequence of these actions is represented by the countless patients suffering chronic pain previously managed successfully by judicious use of opioids who were obliged to seek other sources for relief. Many turned to criminal enterprises, where opioids are often available at prices less than that of prescription drugs. Finding themselves dependent upon an opioid of uncertain composition, the patient is thus exposed to a greater risk of lethal overdose from heroin or a mixture of heroin and fentanyl. Indeed, while some have celebrated a decrease in overdose deaths from prescription opioids as a sign of the success of more stringent prescribing habits, that decrease has been more than balanced by an increased number of deaths due to illicit opioids; the total number of deaths continues to rise. How many occur in patients turned away from legitimate sources is unknown.

SUPPRESSION OF OPIUM CULTIVATION

John Walters, director from 2001 to 2009 of the Office of National Drug Control Policy, believed that a solution to our heroin problem could be found in suppression of cultivation of the opium poppy.[31] Afghanistan, source of 90% of the total world output, was a prime target. In addition to manual destruction of the crop, aerial spraying with toxic herbicides was employed. The efforts did little but poison the populace and alienate the Afghan farmers dependent on the crop for income.

New crops were quickly planted to replace those destroyed. In 2014, 553,000 acres were devoted to opium cultivation, a 43% increase over 2012.[32] Much of the heroin derived therefrom would reach the United States. But what if we could eliminate Afghanistan as a source of opium? Alas, the poppy is a hardy flower able to be grown on the majority of the land surface of the planet. Given the billions of dollars in profits to be made, eradication in one region would quickly be followed by flourishing production elsewhere.

If we cannot control the cultivation of the opium poppy and the production of heroin, perhaps we can stop the entry of opioids into our country by sealing the borders. In fictional accounts of heroin trafficking, we have become accustomed to hearing the weight of smuggled heroin expressed in a metric unit, the kilogram, 1,000 grams. Converted to English units, a kilo is equal to 2.2 pounds. And this brings us to the subject of drug potency.

DRUG POTENCY AND THE LIFE OF THE SMUGGLER

The common English definition of *potency* is the power or the ability to bring about a particular effect. In pharmacology, the meaning is more precise and somewhat different: Potency refers to the *quantity* of a drug required to produce an effect. Thus, while it often is said that heroin is more powerful than morphine, the real meaning is that heroin is the more potent, in the pharmacological sense, of the two drugs. For example, to achieve equally effective relief of severe pain, the intravenous dose of morphine required is about three times greater than that of heroin; put another way, heroin is three times more potent than morphine. This difference in potency matters not at all to the patient in pain; both drugs provide relief. But to the smuggler, potency is very important.

Drug mules are people who crosses borders with illicit drugs strapped to their bodies or even hidden within their bodies. The latter technique involves filling small balloons with a drug such as heroin, swallowing the balloons, and retrieving the drug after crossing the border. Potency is important: for heroin versus morphine, it means 3 balloons instead of 10 for the same number of doses. Fentanyl, a synthetic opioid responsible for thousands of deaths in the United States, is about 30 times as potent as heroin. The fentanyl equivalent of 1 kilo of heroin weighs 30 grams, about the weight of a double-A battery. A relative of fentanyl, carfentanil, has recently begun to arrive in West Virginia, Ohio, and elsewhere, where it has already been responsible for several deaths. Carfentanil is about 5,000 times more potent than heroin. That means that instead of a kilo of heroin, the smuggler need only bring in carfentanil with the weight of an average raindrop. Heroin mules will soon be history only to be replaced by the services of UPS, FedEx, DHL, and the US Postal Service. The advent of drugs such as fentanyl and carfentanil has made securing our borders against opioids exponentially more difficult; impossible, some might argue. No physical wall will keep them out.

THE ROLE OF EDUCATION: JUST SAY NO

Over the past five decades or so, many observers have concluded that a significant reduction in the supply of illicit opioids is unattainable and, recognizing that supply follows demand, have sought means to reduce the latter. The goal is admirable. Professors Avram Goldstein of Stanford University and Harold Kalant of the University of Toronto put it this way: A reduced demand for drugs offers the only real hope of eventually achieving, not a drug-free society, but one with substantially less drug abuse.[33] But the means to that goal are problematic. In 1988, the Justice Department's view, echoed to this day, is that prosecution of drug users is the most effective way to reduce demand.

Much hope has been placed in the efficacy of education in reducing demand for psychoactive drugs. Indeed, in a book published in 2009, John Walters, noted earlier as an advocate of crop eradication, expressed the view that all drug abuse is a consequence of "moral poverty," which could be corrected through "religion and education."[34]

At several points in this book, I have mentioned Cochrane reviews as the gold standard for the evaluation of medical interventions. In examining the role of education in reducing demand for illicit drugs, the Cochrane group evaluated 23 studies, which included nearly 200,000 young people exposed to mass media campaigns between 1991 and 2012. Their summary: "Overall the available evidence does not allow conclusions about the effect of media campaigns on illicit drug use among young people."[35] Despite the expenditure of billions of dollars, we remain uncertain of the efficacy of slogans such as Nancy Reagan's Just Say No, programs such as Drug Abuse Resistance Education (DARE), and advertisements such as "Your Brain on Drugs." Certainly, there is no place for patently dishonest "education" as seen in the 1930s *Reefer Madness*. This is not to say that education cannot work but only that we have not yet figured out how to make it work as a means to significantly reduce demand for opioids.

PLEASURE AND PREJUDICE

In most discussions of how demand for opioids might be reduced, there are, I believe, not one but two elephants in the room. The first is the failure to acknowledge the fact that drugs, including opioids, can bring pleasure defined in the broadest of terms. It can be in John Jones's comment in 1700 that opium causes "a most delicious and extraordinary refreshment of the spirits . . ." or De Quincey, a century later, citing "a respite . . . from the secret burdens of the heart." Drug-induced pleasure can also take the form of the delight which follows relief from torment, whether that torment be physical pain or the much more subtle torments induced by despair. This pleasure seeking is not, as Michael Kinsley pointed out many years ago, confined to a small self-destructive minority but is shared by the most boring and respectable citizens.[36] To the pharmacological puritan, today's seeking of drug-induced pleasure is sinful. Others regard it as the modern manifestation of a search begun by the earliest humans. It is often said that prohibition of alcohol by the 18th Amendment failed because of the rise of crime and corruption associated with it. More convincing is the argument that repeal came about because Americans like the pleasures of alcohol.

If abolition of the human drive to seek pleasure seems unlikely, the second elephant to which I alluded is at least susceptible to pragmatic intervention. I refer to the social factors which drive individuals to seek the comfort provided by opium and her daughters. Significant among the multiple roots of opioid addiction are poverty, unemployment, and social inequities. These have long been present in our inner cities and, more recently, have appeared in areas of the country where meaningful employment in mining, manufacturing, and farming has been reduced. The full impact of robots and other products of artificial intelligence on the employment opportunities of the minimally educated has yet to be seen. Correlations between unemployment and recent epidemics of opioid and methamphetamine addiction are not only mathematically significant but also likely to be causative. In addition to the despair due to these tangible factors, we have self-medication of untreated anxiety, depression, and psychosis arising from deficits in what have come to be given, in the context of our gun epidemic, the umbrella term "mental health." Carl Hart, professor of neuroscience and psychology at Columbia University, has written eloquently of the role of racial injustice as both a driver of opioid addiction and a barrier to effective treatment.[37] Whether our society can at some point acknowledge the dishonesty of ignoring these factors remains to be seen. More important, have we the political will to correct them?

HARM REDUCTION

Recognition of the reality that the supply of opioids from drug cartels is not likely to diminish and that demand by Americans for these drugs is steady if not increasing, we must turn to efforts to reduce the harm done, including death, in those already addicted; those who suffer from what is now enshrined in *The Diagnostic and Statistical Manual of Mental Disorders* of the American Psychiatric Society as "opioid use disorder." Collectively, these efforts are referred to as harm reduction. A number of these were discussed in chapter 2. Prominent among them is access to the opioid antagonist, naloxone (Narcan). Widespread education about and availability of naloxone to reverse opioid overdoses has become routine. More and more communities are equipping their police, firefighters, and other first responders with naloxone. Some have suggested that naloxone be made available over the counter and in place in every home where an opioid is present.

Needle exchange programs have been proven to reduce the risk of infection with HIV and hepatitis B and C due to the sharing of dirty needles. Carrying this pragmatic approach further is the provision of supervised injection sites, as discussed in chapter 2. These sites presently exist in more than 60 cities around the world, and it is said that they have never been associated with a death due to overdose. A second indication of benefit comes from Vancouver, British Columbia, where nearly half of those making use of the injection site enter treatment programs. Though much opposed by pharmacological puritans, supervised sites were, in 2018, being considered in San Francisco, Baltimore, Seattle, Philadelphia, and New York City. My feelings were nicely expressed by a staff writer at the *Economist* magazine: "It takes guts to legalize drugs when so many are dying from them. But it is better that addicts take safe doses of familiar substances under sanitary conditions than for them to risk their lives enriching criminals."[38] I am reminded of a suggestion made nearly a half century ago by Lewis Thomas, a distinguished American physician, medical school dean, and writer.

> The thing to do is to get rid of (the illicit heroin industry), and one way to do it is to put the government into the center of it as an unbeatable competitor. The methadone maintenance program . . . should take us at least part of the way there. There are a great many addicts who have wearied of their way of life and wish to give it up before they are killed by it; most of these are in their twenties, and the record already establishes that a majority of this group can be successfully rescued by methadone. For them, the joy has already gone out of heroin, and the main business of the day is to raise enough cash to buy the heroin that will keep them from withdrawal sickness. If all addicts could be put on methadone, the market would collapse . . . [39]

Dr. Thomas then boldly went on to suggest, and recall that this was 50 years ago, the provision of heroin in a government program for those few not ready to give up the pleasures of the drug. As offensive as is the thought of such programs to the pharmacological puritan, we saw in chapter 2 how heroin maintenance has been applied in Canada since 2005. From experience in Canada and in multiple European programs of heroin maintenance, beneficial effects have been observed in retaining users in treatment, improved social function both in employment and in family life, and a reduction in drug-related crime.

OPIOID REPLACEMENT THERAPY: A TERRIBLE PERVERSION?

Despite Dr. Thomas's long ago endorsement of methadone maintenance as a form of opioid replacement therapy (ORT), there is no aspect of opioid addiction treatment which more clearly marks the divide between pharmacological puritans and nonideological pragmatists. The World Health Organization has called ORT the most promising method of reducing the harm done by drug dependence. Yet, when an expansion of methadone maintenance in New York City was proposed in 1998, the then mayor, Rudolph Giuliani, said that this was a "terrible, terrible perversion of drug treatment" and would only make more people "addicted to methadone which is perhaps a worse addiction."[40] The addition of buprenorphine to ORT in 2002 has done nothing to suppress such ignorance. In 2017, during his 231-day tenure as secretary of Health and Human Services, Tom Price, in disparaging ORT, said that methadone is simply "substituting one opioid for another."[41] His failure to distinguish between physical dependence and addiction or to acknowledge the role of ORT in successful treatment programs is remarkable in a University of Michigan–trained physician. Unfortunately, such remarks regarding ORT have made their way into our judicial system.

Drug courts came into being in the 1980s in response to increasing use of cocaine and the recognition by some that imprisonment was not an efficacious treatment for drug addiction. As an alternative to incarceration, the offender was obliged to report to the court regularly and remain drug-free. Soon the idea was expanded to include users of opioids. However, to this day, nearly all opioid drug courts, like Mr. Guiliani and Dr. Price, reject the use of ORT. Instead, they require detoxification as I described to you in chapter 2; over a period of 14 days, the opioid dose is gradually decreased to zero, thus ameliorating the withdrawal syndrome. The fact is that this imposition of drug abstinence, however attractive it may be to pharmacological puritans, has repeatedly been shown to be less efficacious than ORT in treating opioid addiction. Similar detoxification is imposed on physically dependent persons upon their entry into prison.

Treatment considerations aside, there is an unintended consequence of court or prison-imposed detoxification. Upon leaving prison or court supervision, the detoxified individual is no longer pharmacologically tolerant to opioids. With this loss in tolerance, the risk of overdose death is significantly increased if there is a return to the predetoxification dose of heroin, fentanyl, or prescription opioid.[42]

A VIEW FROM THE TRENCHES

So far we have considered ORT in rather abstract terms. Audrey M. Provenzano has provided a personal account. Dr. Provenzano, a graduate of the Yale University School of Medicine, is now a primary care physician associated with the Massachusetts General Hospital and Harvard Medical School. In 2018, she wrote an article on ORT which appeared in the *New England Journal of Medicine*.[43]

In it, she described a patient, Ms. L., who came regularly to her office, usually in the company of her granddaughter. But one day she appeared alone, clearly agitated and in tears. Ms. L. confessed that years ago she had been an opioid addict, drug-free for decades, but that she had recently relapsed using her husband's oxycodone pills. Her greatest fear was that her family would discover her secret and that she would be cut off from her granddaughter.

Wanting only "to feel normal again," Ms. L. asked that Dr. Provenzano prescribe buprenorphine. But Dr. Provenzano could not because she had not taken the brief training required to prescribe that drug. In fact, she did not wish to deal with patients needing ORT; she had heard too many stories of the difficulties of treating those with opioid use disorder. Instead, she referred Ms. L. to a colleague. Ms. L. stopped meeting her appointments with Dr. Provenzano. A year passed and then one evening she learned that Ms. L. had died of an opioid overdose.

Dr. Provenzano is a modest woman, and she does not flatter herself that she could have saved Ms. L. But, facing the shame that she felt, she reminded herself that she had had a trusting relationship with Ms. L. and that perhaps she could have made a difference. "She had trusted me. And I turned her away." Subsequently, Dr. Provenzano acquired the waiver to prescribe buprenorphine and now treats a group of patients suffering opioid use disorder. She now realizes that such individuals frequently have, in addition to addiction, complex social and behavioral needs often requiring a team approach. But it is opioid replacement, in the form of buprenorphine, which permits the journey to recovery to begin. In her closing paragraph, Dr. Provenzano says this:

> Caring for these patients has become the most meaningful part of my practice. . . . Providing some sense of normalcy for patients whose lives are roiled by overdose and estrangement is the most profound therapeutic intervention I've engaged in as a caregiver. I did not know what Ms. L. meant all those years ago when she said that she only wanted to feel normal again. I wish that I'd listened more closely. I wish that I had not been afraid.

WE HAVE MET THE ENEMY

For the pharmacological puritan, drug-induced pleasure, or at least that not involving nicotine or alcohol, is sinful; one cannot be flexible with sin. Nor is a rational approach available to those unable to perceive differences between what we call drugs of abuse. Dogmatic individuals, however well intentioned, can only hinder our progress toward a sane balance between individual freedom and the pursuit of happiness on the one hand and, on the other, our society's obligation to protect its members, especially the young, from harm.

I will close this chapter with the words of Walt Kelly's Pogo Possum.

We have met the enemy and he is us.

NOTES

1. Mencken HL, Cooke A (1990) *The Vintage Mencken.* New York: Vintage.
2. Yost P (1988) Prosecute drug users to shut off demand, Justice Department urges. *New York Times* A-9, March 20.
3. Bennett W (1990) Should drugs be legalized? *Readers Digest* 165:90–97.
4. Sessions JB (2016) Senate Caucus on International Narcotics Control SD-226, April 5.
5. Teter CJ, McCabe SE, Cranford JA, Boyd CJ, Guthrie SK (2005) Prevalence and motives for illicit use of prescription simulants in an undergraduate sample. *J Am Coll Health* 53(6):253–262.
6. Nutt D (2012) Drugs are taken for pleasure—Realize this and we can start to reduce harm. *The Guardian*, December 3.
7. The Doctrine and Covenants of The Church of Jesus Christ of Latter-day Saints Containing Revelations Given to Joseph Smith (1833). https://www.lds.org/scriptures/dc-testament?lang=eng
8. United Nations Office on Drugs and Crime (2018) The International Drug Control Conventions. https://www.unodc/documents/commissions/CND/Int

9. Fisher G (2014) The Drug War at 100. *Stanford Lawyer*, December 19.

10. Udell GG (1972) *Opium and Narcotic Laws*. Washington, D.C.: U.S. Government Printing Office.

11. Leary v. United States, 395 U.S. 6 (1969) Justia › US Law › US Case Law › US Supreme Court › Volume 395 › Leary v. United States

12. Nixon RM (1971) Remarks about an intensified program for drug abuse prevention and control. June 17. www.presidency.ucsb.edu/ws/?pid=3047

13. Baum D (2016) Legalize it all. *Harper's Magazine*. https://harpers.org/archive/2016/04/legalize-it-all/

14. Congress of the United States (1986) Anti-Drug Abuse Act of 1986. https://www.congress.gov/bill/99th-congress/house-bill/5484

15. New York Civil Liberties Union (2009) The Rockefeller drug laws: Unjust, irrational, ineffective https://www.nyclu.org/en/.../rockefeller-drug-laws-unjust-irrational-ineffective-2009

16. Editorial (2010) A new dawn for drug policy in the USA. *The Lancet* 375(9728):1754.

17. United States Department of Justice (2013) Memorandum for all United States Attorneys: Guidance regarding marijuana enforcement. August 29. https://www.justice.gov/iso/opa/resources/3052013829132756857467.pdf

18. Congress of the United States (2016) H.Amdt.332 to Commerce, Justice, Science, and Related Agencies Appropriations Act, H.R. 2578. https://www.congress.gov/amendment/114th-congress/house-amendment/332

19. Centers for Disease Control and Prevention (2017) Drug overdose death data. https://www.cdc.gov/drugoverdose/data/statedeaths.html

20. AZ Quotes (2018) Baruch Spinoza. https://www.azquotes.com/quote/500072

21. Ferreira S (2017) Portugal's radical drugs policy is working. Why hasn't the world copied? *The Guardian*, December 5.

22. Holder E (2017) *The Hill*, October 10. https://thehill.com/

23. Marks R, Sachar E (1973) Undertreatment of medical inpatients with narcotic analgesics. *Ann Intern Med* 78(2):173–181.

24. Phillips D (2000) JCAHO pain management standards are unveiled. Joint Commission on Accreditation of Healthcare Organizations. *JAMA* 284(4):428–429.

25. Porter J, Jick H (1980) Addiction rare in patients treated with narcotics. *NEJM* 302:123.

26. Meier B (2018) *Pain Killer: An Empire of Deceit and the Origin of America's Opioid Epidemic*. New York: Random House.

27. United States Department of Justice (2017) Founder and owner of pharmaceutical company *Insys* arrested and charged with racketeering. https://www.justice.gov/opa/pr/founder-and-owner-pharmaceutical-company-insys-arrested-and-charged-racketeering

28. United States Attorney's Office, Southern District of New York (2018) Five Manhattan doctors indicted for accepting bribes and kickbacks from a pharmaceutical company in exchange for prescribing powerful fentanyl narcotic. https://www.justice.gov/.../five-manhattan-doctors-indicted-accepting-bribes-and-kick

29. Dowell D, Haegerich TM, Shou R (2016) CDC Guidelines for prescribing opioids for chronic pain—United States, 2016. *JAMA* 315(15):1624–1645.

30. Martin SA, Potee RA, Lazris A (2016) Neat, plausible, and generally wrong: A response to the CDC recommendations for chronic opioid use. https://medium.com/@stmartin/neat-plausible-and-generally-wrong-a-response-to-the-cdc-recommendations-for-chronic-opioid-use-5c9d9d319f71

31. Straziuso J (2007) Afghanistan won't spray poppy plants. *Washington Post*, January 25. www.washingtonpost.com/wp-dyn/content/article/2007/01/25/AR2007012500435.html

32. United Nations Office on Drugs and Crime (2014) Afghanistan Opium Survey 2014. Cultivation and production. https://www.unodc.org/documents/crop-monitoring/Afghanistan/Afghan-opium-survey-2014.pdf

33. Goldstein A, Kalant H (1990) Drug policy: Striking the right balance. *Science* 249(4976):1513–1521.

34. Dililio JJ, Walters JP, Bennett W (1996) *Body Count: Moral Poverty . . . And How to Win America's War Against Crime and Drugs.* New York: Simon & Schuster.

35. Allara E, Ferri M, Bo A, Gasparrini A, Faggiano F (2015) Are mass-media campaigns effective in preventing drug use? A Cochrane systematic review and meta-analysis. *BMJ Open* 3;5(9):e007449. doi:10.1136/bmjopen-2014-007449.

36. Kinsley M (1988) Glass houses and getting stoned. *Time*, June 6.

37. Hart C (2013). *High Price.* New York: Harper Collins.

38. Anonymous (2017) *The Economist*, May 20: 17–18.

39. Thomas L (1972) Notes of a biology watcher—heroin. *NEJM* 286:531–533.

40. Ciment J (1998) Clash in US over methadone treatment. *The Lancet* 252:1205.

41. Kaplan S (2018) F.D.A. to expand medication-assisted therapy for opioid addicts. *The New York Times*, February 25.

42. Strang J, McCambridge J, Best D, Beswick T, Bearn J, Rees S, Gossop M (2003) Loss of tolerance and overdose mortality after in patient opiate detoxification: A follow-up study. *BMJ* 326:959–960.

43. Provenzano AM (2018) Caring for Ms. L.—Overcoming my fear of treating opioid use disorder. *NEJM* 78(7):600–601.

INDEX

For the benefit of digital users, indexed terms that span two pages (e.g., 52–53) may, on occasion, appear on only one of those pages.